The Consumer Handbook on Hearing Loss and Hearing Aids

A Bridge to Healing

CHAPTERS RECOMMENDED BY YOUR HEARING HEALTH CARE PROVIDER

Dedication

To all who seek a better way.

The Consumer Handbook on Hearing Loss and Hearing Aids

A Bridge to Healing

Edited by
Clinical Audiologist
Dr. Richard Carmen

Auricle Ink Publishers • Sedona, Arizona

Library of Congress Cataloging in Publication Data

Carmen, Richard
    The Consumer Handbook on Hearing Loss and Hearing Aids:
    A Bridge to Healing
    Auricle Ink Publishers
    1. Hearing loss—Popular works. 2. Hearing disorders.
    3. Hearing problems. 4. Hearing aids.
    RF290.C373 1998   617.8'9   97-77946

Third Printing

ISBN 0-9661826-0-X

Cover Photo: Rio Grande Gorge by Bela Kalman
Cover Layout by Richard Drayton

Auricle Ink Publishers
P.O.Box 20607, Sedona AZ 86341
(520) 284-0860
www.hearingproblems.com

TABLE OF CONTENTS

Foreword

Donna L. Sorkin
Executive Director
Self Help for Hard of Hearing People [SHHH]
Bethesda, Maryland

Congratulations! Having found this book, you've now taken that first critical step toward living better with hearing loss, that of educating yourself about what you need to do to improve your communication. Although you may never have normal hearing again, with today's advanced hearing technology and with some changes in how you approach communication, you can learn to function effectively in a variety of settings. For easy previewing of chapter material, I recommend reading each of the four Section Introductions. This will allow you, in a page or two, to see the content of what follows.

When my own hearing began to change nearly 20 years ago, I was a young woman with a family, friends and a challenging career. I knew very little about hearing loss other than it was causing me considerable apprehension and some problems in communicating on the job and in noisy situations. I was embarrassed—no, I was actually mortified—that this was happening to me! My competent and caring audiologist told me that I needed hearing aids. But like most people, I had preconceived and incorrect notions about them, and minimal understanding of the complexity of hearing loss itself. I also had literally no guidance to help me adjust to the emotional and functional impact of not hearing properly. I can say that, fortunately, much has changed since that time.

Hearing health care professionals, educators, and consumers like you and me, increasingly recognize that providing information and support to people with hearing loss is crucial to living successfully with it. The wonderful original work in this book, written by the best of professionals the field of hearing health care offers, achieves its goal of, once again, gaining control of your life.

My own search for information and support led me to the organization with which I am now associated, the largest membership organization in the world for people with hearing loss. SHHH* seeks to provide educational outreach to an estimated 28 million people with hearing loss in the United States. We know firsthand from thousands of letters we receive each year that people with hearing loss do not have

*For more information on SHHH, see their listing in Chapter 14.

the same access to educational materials typically available to those with other health-related problems. They want resources like this book, and up-to-date information on the latest technology, employability concerns, legal issues, and more.

The body of work assembled in this book by clinical audiologist and educator Richard Carmen, covers wide-ranging topics of interest to hard of hearing people and their families. All chapters were authored by audiologists who work on a daily basis with hard of hearing people. Much material covers hearing aids, such as selection and care, fundamental subjects for anyone with loss of hearing. At the same time, although hearing aids are the single most important therapeutic factor in addressing hearing loss, your efforts to overcome the challenge of living in the mainstream as a hard of hearing person should not end with the hearing aid purchase. There will frequently be some situations in which you need help by something other than hearing aids. Too often, these devices are given short shrift, but in Chapter 13, you'll discover a range of choices available to you which will pleasantly augment your hearing aids.

As an advocate for people with hearing loss, I personally know that people can help themselves immensely if they know what to expect and the right questions to ask. Further, the most successful hearing aid users are usually people who truly understand the substantial benefits as well as the limitations of amplification. I believe this book will give you the understanding you need in order to come to terms with your hearing loss.

I would add one other general recommendation to the useful guidance found among these many pages. Most people find that even after they've educated themselves and have been given appropriate professional assistance, they benefit enormously from talking with others who understand the same struggles. Consumer organizations, whether national or local, provide opportunities for people to share helpful hints and emotional support. The resources section at the end of this book [Chapter 14] offers a useful listing of organizations which includes many consumer groups specializing in this kind of special care.

Whether you're just beginning the trek along the road to better hearing, or you're already on it and looking for some additional help and direction, your future is promising. Technology continues to improve, and hearing loss is increasingly viewed as a health condition that, like many others, needn't be insurmountable. By taking an active part in your own hearing health care, you'll live an easier life, a less stressful and happier one for you and all who are around you.

Introduction

Section I: Hearing Loss

Karl E. Strom and Marjorie D. Skafte
Editors, *The Hearing Review*
Duluth, Minnesota

Make no mistake about it, hearing loss is serious. Emerging data continues to link and/or associate the most common type of hearing loss, sensorineural, to a variety of physical and psychosocial dysfunctions, isolation, depression, hypertension and stress, dependent living, and even illnesses such as ischemic heart disease and arrhythmia. Perhaps even worse, people who have hearing problems are deprived of some of the most cherished moments in life: the laughter and tender words of a grandchild, easy conversations with friends and companions, and the sounds of nature. Most people who seek hearing help, simply want to hear what they're missing.

People who have hearing loss are certainly not alone. It's estimated that 25-28 million people in the U.S.—or about one in ten individuals—have a significant hearing loss; 120 million people worldwide have hearing loss significant enough to interfere with communication. Studies show that the average male will lose 40 percent of his birthright inner ear hair cells by age of 65. In a lifetime, the causes for such loss may include everything from industrial machinery to fireworks, or howling babies to big bands. In the U.S., perhaps it's no wonder that approximately one million people each year purchase hearing aids, and still others purchase assistive listening devices.

Whatever your questions about hearing loss, you'll find excellent advice and answers in this book which is written by some of the world's most respected members of the hearing health care field. This first section focuses on causes and effects of hearing impairment. It explores the important human side of living with loss of hearing, and the need for taking positive action. You'll find "sound" information about your options.

In Chapter 1, Editor and Clinical Audiologist Richard Carmen explores the emotional obstacles blocking the path of accepting a hearing loss, and your choice to do something about it. He details

3

the wide range of feelings that are common during the "acceptance process," and offers some brief tests that assess the extent to which your hearing might be affecting you and others around you. Chapter 2, written by James F. Maurer, Ph.D., recounts a number of poignant, and often humorous experiences reported to him by adult hearing impaired clients. He strongly advocates taking charge of one's life to solve any hearing problems. In Chapter 3, H. Gustav Mueller, Ph.D., explains the various types of hearing loss, the terminology and factors relating to sound and the auditory system, and debunks 10 myths about hearing loss and hearing aids. Robert E. Sandlin, Ph.D., in Chapter 4, provides practical advice on how to seek professional help. He offers descriptions of the unique qualifications of audiologists and hearing instrument specialists, provides tips on the qualities to look for when selecting a hearing care professional, and describes the various aspects of a hearing assessment.

The cochlea, its hair cells and all the other parts that make up our auditory system are nothing short of a biological marvel. As just one example, hair cell bundles are so sensitive in their detection of sound that one researcher has likened their movements to the top of the Eiffel Tower shifting by only a thumb's width. When you realize that researchers are only now beginning to understand how our ears and brains process sound, it's easy to see why the road to better hearing can, at times, be a bumpy one. Because of the often gradual nature of hearing loss, it's natural for people to have resistance when it comes to taking action in solving their hearing problems. Likewise, hearing aids and other solutions may solve communication problems very effectively, but may not always provide perfect hearing for all listening situations. As with any journey down a bumpy road, the authors' chapters encourage you to become informed about the route, ask for directions along the way, and continue toward the destination of better hearing. We think you'll find much in the book to prepare you for this journey.

CHAPTER ONE

The Emotions of Losing Hearing and a Bridge to Healing

Richard Carmen, Au.D.

Dr. Carmen recently received his Doctor of Audiology Degree from the Arizona School of Health Sciences,a division of the Kirksville College of Osteopathic Medicine. He's been practicing audiology and issuing hearing aids for more than 25 years, during which time he pioneered research into the effects of metabolic diseases on hearing. He has authored two previous consumer books, *Our Endangered Hearing: Understanding and Coping with Hearing Loss* (1977), and *Positive Solutions to Hearing Loss* (1983). As former Editor-in-Chief of *Hear,* a Southern California consumer Newsletter, he published more than 100 articles by contributing professionals on topics related to hearing problems. He's been a Consultant to the Legal Services Unit of the California Department of Consumer Affairs, taught university graduate classes in Audiology, and currently maintains a small practice among the red rocks of Sedona, Arizona.

As Quasimodo, the Hunchback of Notre Dame, lay dying in the arms of the beautiful gypsy girl La Esmeralda, a tear rolls down his cheek. In his dying moment, he realizes his greatest torment—the pain of feeling. He whispers to Esmeralda, "Why could I not have been made of stone?"

Feelings and emotions characterize us as human beings. To feel at all is a risk. This emotional experience may be wonderful, painful, and sometimes perplexing. Yet, more than our physical body, feelings are the substance of our identity. Each of us reacts differently toward the varied experiences of our lives. For centuries, fields of study have been devoted to exploring this fascinating phenomena, but the search has yielded remarkably little knowledge. Therefore, I broach this topic carefully and with reservation.

A university professor of mine once said to me in graduate school, "You can explore the HOW'S and WHAT'S of a problem but don't ever try to solve the question WHY because it can't be scientifically answered." And here I am writing a chapter which in part addresses why you may be feeling a particular emotion (emotion no less!) and what to do about it. Nevertheless, from three decades of clinical practice, I've observed some interesting emotions and feelings in my patients. These observations extend into my own family members with loss of hearing, so I not only have firsthand clinical experience of the feelings we'll be talking about here, they also deeply touch home. I believe it's important to know what we feel. Maybe that's why I married a psychologist! Hopefully, this chapter will help you and your family understand the feelings about hearing loss, and what might be done about it.

I taught a course once in which I had my students wear earplugs for a full day—morning to bedtime. They were asked to log every feeling and emotion they went through and report to the class the following week. We all were overwhelmed by two things: the experiences from student to student were similar, and their emotions ran deeply about their experiences.

Students said they felt inadequate and incompetent. There was a sense of limitation in areas they'd taken for granted. Simple tasks like using the telephone couldn't be performed without special focus, difficulty or strain. Common sounds like ice stirred in a glass, running water, or the page of a book being turned, which orient us in our environment, had suddenly faded or disappeared altogether. Driving the car took on a whole new experience. With the absence of wind and traffic, there was a feeling of disorientation. Students quickly realized how important their vision became to compensate for what they could not hear, and even that wasn't enough.

By the end of the day most of the students confessed they were unnerved and depressed. One student reported she had collapsed into bed crying. I believe their collective reactions were directly linked to feelings of inadequacy—a deficiency in their daily performance relative to how they were used to functioning. Once the earplugs were removed, all students felt relieved. Their sense of normalcy and calm returned. I remember another student in particular saying, "What a horrible experience!" An apt description.

While this experiment was useful to normal hearing students, it revealed what you no doubt already know. Hearing is an essential human sense. Its absence would be greatly missed by anyone. And as hearing declines, similar to other sensory deficits, we humans have an extraordinary ability to compensate for the loss. Such compensation is a built-in defense mechanism to which we give little thought. It just happens. If you survive a heart attack, the body works quickly to establish other arteries and connections. If you lose your sense of smell, your eyes become more probing. If vision goes, hearing often sharpens. And when hearing deteriorates, an array of latent abilities kick in. When they do, the act of compensation can fool you. You may do well for awhile with partial hearing loss, and not even recognize its presence. You might cast it off as poor attention, for example. It's for this reason that loss of hearing gives the impression of being so insidious. "It just kind of crept up on me!" most hearing health care professionals hear from their patients. Of course it didn't really creep up. It's just that early suspicions went ignored.

Something you've probably said many times in your life, and will see repeated, rephrased and re-analyzed in this book, is the complaint, "I hear but I don't understand the words clearly!" This is particularly true when trying to communicate in a group, around a few people, or in an environment with background noise such as in a restaurant or automobile. Early on, when you had problems hearing, you may have passed it off as being no more troublesome for you than for anyone else in the same situation. But as issues around poor hearing grew more apparent and the process of communication began breaking down, you must have realized the problem was not going away.

People who develop hearing loss from an explosion, accident, or other trauma are probably more inclined to deal with it because it is sudden and readily apparent. But if you're in generally good health and are the type of person who doesn't like to think of yourself as less capable than anyone else, you may have started blaming other people for frequent mis-communication. Typically, you may think others are not speaking clearly or loudly enough, or that they "mumble" their words. It's only when sufficient numbers of people close to you suggest that it's <u>you</u> and not them, you get your first inkling of something within your personal communication system has gone awry. Some people never come to this realization and go on believing that others are the source of their communication failure. They continue to blame and be angry.

Our ego is attached to our health. We like to think of ourselves as being in shape, with a good heart, teeth, bones, vision—and good hearing. To resist the reality of hearing loss perpetuates mis-communication and the emotions that go with not hearing well. If we try to ignore it, or stop thinking about it, the problem doesn't go away. For some people, the crossroads of acknowledging hearing difficulty and doing something about it is the point where they vacillate so much, they end up doing nothing. The process of deciding to do something may take years. In the meantime, the problem becomes compounded. A host of feelings can reign, from suppression and projection to denial. In the end, none of them serve one's health.

Let's look at examples of how feelings may affect the way you perceive solutions. "Hearing difficulties" pertain to specific situations (like trying to hear someone speaking to you). A "hearing problem" is your internalization, or how you process the issues surrounding these situations (like getting angry at people if you can't hear them). These terms are often mistakenly interchanged. If you're in the living room watching television with your family and you realize that you're missing too much dialogue, you might ask others in the room if you can turn the volume louder, in which case you think you've solved the difficulty.

The reality is that undoubtedly your family will object to having the television too loud. This may make you feel angry, resentful, embarrassed, guilty, selfish, annoyed or any other ill feeling—and it's a sure sign of a hearing problem. You're internalizing feelings about a hearing difficulty. This is neither healthy nor in your best interest. The first step in solving these difficulties is to acknowledge how you feel about your hearing loss. A willingness to consider it a fact of life will create a solid bridge to healing. It's the foundation upon which all hearing problems find resolution.

There are two common philosophies people seem to adopt once hearing loss has become a part of their lives: you can try to cover up the fact that you have it, or you can tell others when the occasion is appropriate that you don't hear well. There are many variations between both themes but if you're willing to take a close and honest look at yourself, you'll recognize in which direction you're more polarized.

The emotions a person feels when hearing loss is confirmed takes the full gamut of human experiences. Some are relieved that at last they know that this is the cause of their problem. Others are horrified—it seems an unbelievable possibility that the problem could be wholly theirs. Each of us have our own specific internal (feelings) and external (people around us) influences, such that predicting how we might respond to the news of having impaired hearing becomes quite complex. Furthermore, your reactions to hearing loss do not necessarily equate to the degree of impairment; that is, you can have a mild loss of hearing which impacts your life more profoundly than someone with greater loss. Your reactions will be most influenced by how you feel about yourself and the world around you, and how other people close to you react to your problem.

Denying Hearing Loss

If your hearing health care provider informs you that you have an irreversible loss, which happens to be the most common type, you may not want to hear this news. On the other hand, if you don't believe it, you're probably pushing the envelope of denial. One of the first questions I'm asked in my practice from someone who has real trouble accepting hearing loss is typically, "Is it reversible?" "Is there surgery for it?" "It won't get too much worse, will it?" While these questions may indicate some denial, the truth is, only on extremely rare occasions are patients seen in full denial. It's more often a matter that, yes, the hearing loss was always suspected, but, it wasn't the news they wanted and they'd rather push it out of their minds.

Denial is the rejection of what's really happening to your body. Often, it provides a useful function by allowing you time to recover from the initial shock. But some trap themselves here for years and others for a lifetime. Denial is an act of concealment, and sometimes the ultimate deception to oneself. To deny the notion of hearing loss is to claim that you are all right, in good health, perhaps still "perfect." But none of us is really perfect, are we?

If you're a person wondering if you're experiencing denial as you continue reading here—likely not. You probably wouldn't be reading this book otherwise (although you could read it and say, "That's not me he's talking about!"). If you're well aware of the loss, but deny its presence when others inquire, this isn't denial. It's concealment. So, congratulations! At least you're willing to look at the problem. And this often is where a fork in the road appears. Some choose to continue on in life with concealment; others choose to do something about the problem.

By now you must have discovered that your loss is more or less noticeable to you and others depending on circumstances. For example, you may do well on the telephone but need the television turned louder; or your hearing is fine when one person speaks but you miss some of what's being said in a small group. What appears to be inconsistent hearing difficulties may lead others to think you sometimes "selectively listen," and other times, you don't, or that you don't care. Worse yet, it can fool you! You may cast it off as poor acoustics in the room, or "people mumble."

Because hearing loss is often gradual over several years, you've probably found ways to compensate by telling yourself, "People just need to speak up and I'll hear great!"—but, do you really? Or you might interact with others by turning up the TV which solves the problem for you—but what's it done to your family? These denial mechanisms can become an integral way for you to operate in the world. The more sophisticated and highly developed these compensatory responses, the easier it becomes for you to deny the problem.

For example, maybe you have everyone else do the work of helping you hear, like allowing others to repeat, rephrase, speak up and so forth. And you think this solves your problem. Without realizing it, you may even grow skilled at watching a speaker's lips, repeating what you think you hear (to confirm the information), tuning one person out and another in, reducing background noises, making educated guesses, watching facial movements and expressions as well as gestures and body language. These are all excellent and necessary ways to help you hear better and understand more, but the irony is, you can get stuck believing that this is all you need to do. The truth is, this is just the beginning.

Isolation and Avoidance

As we age and begin to lose longtime friends and loved ones, we find ourselves more isolated. Impaired hearing only adds to this isolation, and compounds matters. The experience of separation from others is not limited to the 50+ crowd. I've seen many patients in their 20s and 30s give up their favorite activities because they're unable to hear adequately. I've seen high school students refuse to wear hearing aids because they fear peer ridicule, choosing to be left alone and miss out on social interaction.

When you're isolated, you cut yourself off from the world around you and from the people you love. You avoid situations you know will be difficult; you become a victim of the decision to do nothing to resolve your dilemma; and you're willing to risk the consequences. "No, you go ahead without me," can become a favorite expression. Unable to hear and being isolated is a heartbreaking, painful and lonely way to exist. In centuries, even decades past, when amplification had not yet been developed as we now know it, people had no alternatives, and suffered the consequences of lesser technology. Today, to suffer the consequences is a choice.

The longer you avoid seeking professional help, the more you may fall into other avoidance patterns, and become entrenched with a hearing loss which rules your life. You will find yourself missing the

10

things that mean the most—friends; telephone conversations; family gatherings; dinner parties; card games; theaters; and on and on. *These are the pleasures of life!* They are vital to soothing our nerves, helping us feel nurtured and wanted, and keeping us intellectually stimulated. You must hold onto these pleasures with your most enduring grip.

Frustration and Defeat

In any family where a member has impaired hearing, you'll also find frustration. A frequently heard comment by the person with hearing loss, as well as the family is "I can't stand it anymore!" In fact, the longer the avoidance of hearing loss goes on, often, the greater the frustrations. Communication depends on aural cues. Once this system begins to break down, frustration usually spreads into the lives of the entire family.

For someone who doesn't have hearing loss, it's almost impossible to conceive of this problem. After all, there's no outward sign—no tumor on the head, no fractured joints, no walker in the hand. All anyone observes is the <u>effect</u> of hearing loss, not the hearing loss itself, and it may be glossed over as no big deal.

In addition to frustration, it's easy to feel defeated and not know what else to do. You struggle to hear despite how attentive you are. You're playing an odds game—sooner or later you're going to miss some conversation. Defeat could be your fate if no help was available. Not taking advantage of professional help is not defeat, <u>it's self-defeat</u>. It is resignation, concession, submission, abdication and surrender. This does nothing to lessen the problem.

(If you already wear hearing aids and feel defeated, explore all other options available to you, *many included in this book.*)

Anger

People who are angry over hearing loss have a right to be angry. It is such a vital sense to lose, and its loss influences almost every aspect of socialization. Every time you ask someone to repeat themselves, it's a reminder to you of the problem. It gets stored in a memory bank of the brain. And it just doesn't go away! Eventually, you can become resentful and angry at others over your own need to have things repeated. Worse yet, you may become angry when a family member suggests you should get help. You already know that, you just don't want to hear it from them. It's just too painful.

The dynamics of this emotion can be fairly simple. You may

11

become angry that you're not understood by your spouse or family. The family is upset that this "stubborn person" isn't doing more about the hearing loss. Some hearing impaired people, resistant to the impact their hearing loss has on others, may ask to have things repeated in a blaming manner. This leads others to feel that the communication problem extends *to them* and gets them angry!

You may find that you're as angry with the world as you are with yourself, so it might seem that few people can be trusted to help. Your sense of humor is gone and life seems to have become a great effort. Perhaps you desperately want to make a change but don't know how or where to turn. Indecision like this is a stumbling block that will keep you angry and upset. If you continue ignoring the problem, the issues surrounding it are further perpetuated. If you find solace in reverting to denial of the problem, it's a reprieve—but short-lived—you've already awakened to the truth of your situation. For most people, unexpressed inner turmoil finally shifts from its simmering, hidden view, to boiling over. People around you are less likely to understand from where this hostility arises if you yourself are not in touch with it.

This is terribly wearing on relationships, especially when it's not understood. Once you become attuned that your upset originates from how you feel about yourself (that is, the anger that you carry because of what hearing loss has done to your life), you may discover a renewed sense of calm. Something that nobody may ever have told you, you need to hear: you have a right to be angry! You have a right to cry. You have a right to all your feelings. What's so essential to understand is that directing these emotions to others is likely to fuel the fire.

Selfishness and Resentment

Living with someone who refuses to get help, regardless of the condition, is a challenge. Because the development of hearing loss is typically a slow process, so too, have you probably been having people slowly help you compensate. This sets up a potentially fertile environment for strained family relationships. Your negligence or unwillingness to help yourself may be seen as a selfish act. Of course you're entitled to expect others not to speak to you from another room, or in the presence of such cacophony as a loud television, a vacuum cleaner or stereo. But in the absence of wearing hearing aids, the family shouldn't be expected to manipulate the household for your convenience, especially when it's at the expense of others you care about.

If you're out socially and you're unaided, you already know how fed up your spouse is over seeing you miss conversation. If you're in a movie theater (if in fact you're not avoiding theaters altogether) and your partner or companion must continuously repeat the on-screen dialogue, you might be hearing a lot of "shhh!" from those seated near you. In the meantime, you, your partner and maybe others around you have just missed another line of dialogue.

Rejection

Bill was a likable but boisterous man. He told funny jokes but he told them with such volume that people 30 feet away would laugh. He was a source of constant entertainment as well as embarrassment to his wife and friends. Sitting in a restaurant, he'd talk about people's personal problems. It wasn't that his friends didn't want their problems discussed, they just didn't want the entire restaurant to hear about it. It was as if Bill had no sense of what was appropriate. No one suspected, until I met Bill, his wife and others for lunch one day, that he had a marked loss of hearing. Bill knew it—but he wasn't about to let anyone else in on his secret. His refusal for help cost him the relationships of people who once truly enjoyed and appreciated him. However, his friends simply could no longer tolerate the humiliations that went with the friendship.

Many hearing impaired people are rejected by others who do not know of their affliction. I've seen people accused of suffering from memory difficulties, being disinterested, paranoid, and even senile and stupid, when in fact it was hearing loss. When others remain uninformed about why you may behave or interact the way you do, they're forced to draw wrong conclusions which carry undesirable consequences. It doesn't need to be this way. You don't have to be vulnerable to social rejection. You have to experience this only a few times to know how painful it is.

The Stall

Probably the single most common response that professionals hear from patients, once the presence of hearing loss is explained, is a question posed as emphatically as any statement: "It's not bad enough that I need hearing aids!...Is it?" Such a patient recognizes the presence of the loss but tries to find every excuse not to do anything about it. I call it "the stall." For some, denial may pass as quickly as resolution from anger, but staving off hearing aids requires the expertise of a tight-rope walker—it's a matter of how long you can perpetuate the illusion that you hear when you don't. Surprisingly, some people will lock themselves into procrastination for years. It's the person with hearing loss telling the hearing health care provider, "I'm too young to get hearing aids!" or the spouse being told, "I know I don't hear well, dear, but it's not that bad yet!" Does any of this sound familiar? How about, "We just can't afford it!" or "No one I know likes their hearing aids!" or "Tom has a hearing loss and doesn't wear hearing aids and he gets along just fine—" but, of course, Tom really doesn't.

When someone has made their mind up that they don't want to pursue amplification possibilities, no time is the right time. In the meantime, the world around you can start to fall apart.

Sadness

Helen Keller, both deaf and blind, has said* that if she could have had one sense restored, it would have been her hearing. She believed that hearing keeps us all in the intellectual company of those we love. Vision is not required for intellectual exchange.

The kind of sadness which accompanies hearing loss is not accurately represented as "depression." After all, it's not like you've been told you have a terminal illness and have only six months left. Very few patients ever fall into this kind of "clinical depression" over their hearing loss and then, typically, only with a predisposition for it. On the other hand, it's very common for anyone with impaired hearing to experience a kind of grief. After all, what is there to celebrate? Such feelings are absolutely normal. If you look closely, you may even discover that other family members have shared in your sadness. So often we think that what we feel inside remains hidden there. It's easy to forget that those we love can easily see past this thin veil. And rest assured that they not only see your sadness, but have suffered right along with you. If you doubt this is true—ask them.

The danger of prolonged sadness or grief is that it can eat away at the most meaningful relationships in our lives. It's disabling. It can cost you your vibrant self. It removes the sparkle from your eye and the smile on your face. It's almost like another personality evolves. Unquestionably, people close to you remember the old you before the

*Helen Keller, *Helen Keller in Scotland,* (London: Methuen and Co., 1933)

14

loss, and they want you back. The most effective way to resolve sadness over loss of hearing is by making a positive change. This includes everything from getting hearing aids to using special devices designed to make hearing (and therefore life) easier.

Other Feelings

If you're an average person with hearing loss, you know that your own **impatience** at times has caused you to be harsher than you'd like, or **insensitive, unkind or unfair**. Once you've realized what you've done, you may feel **guilty**. You may wish you could have handled the situation differently but you just couldn't control yourself. You may feel like it's a vicious cycle—you expect loved ones to be your ears, and those around you get **fed up** doing your hearing. No one wins.

When I consult with a hearing impaired person in my office, I always turn to the spouse or companion and ask for his or her feelings about the problem. The common response is, "I'm so **tired** of having to repeat myself!" What isn't said is that everyone feels the same. **Struggling to communicate** under these conditions can be exhausting.

Of the array of emotions you can go through with impaired hearing, something common among almost everyone is **embarrassment**. Second-guessing what you think you hear, offering inappropriate responses, missing the punch line to a joke, or getting wrong directions are small examples of what you and loved ones experience. If you're not comfortable with your communication skills, your subtle cues of **awkwardness** can put others ill at ease.

Statistically and historically, the number one reason people do not wear hearing aids is embarrassment that results from perceived stigma. Ironically, failure to use amplification usually proves to be even more embarrassing. With the advent of the CIC (completely-in-the-canal) hearing aids in the early 1990s, this trend has shifted. The cosmetic appeal of these exceptionally inconspicuous hearing aids have attracted users who would never have considered amplification on any other basis. Hopefully, with continuing technology, embarrassment about hearing aid use will become a thing of the past.

Exploring opportunities in amplification will change your life, and the lives of those you love. In the hearing health care world of today, hearing aids and other appropriate amplification accessories offer anyone with loss of hearing the most efficient avenue to independent hearing. These devices allow you to break free of your dependence on others. Please examine Chapter 13 in this book. These items can make all the difference in strengthening your relationship with those around you rather than fueling unrewarding emotions.

Acceptance and Moving On

It's that easy. Acceptance of hearing loss allows you to move on. You may already recognize the trials and tribulations of inadequate hearing. You may know that despite all efforts to compensate for not hearing, nothing else gets you through. This realization is essential before you can move on with clear vision. Coming to terms with the emotions surrounding your impaired hearing builds a bridge to healing. And acceptance of your hearing loss allows you safe passage across. But before you can move on, you must be honest with yourself.

Expectations versus Actual Performance

If you're a person living in an unamplified world, you no doubt have expectations about hearing which may not align with your ability. I've seen friends of mine with hearing loss refuse to get hearing aids, then go into situations expecting to hear. At the end of the evening, I'd point out how much conversation was missed.

People who haven't yet come to terms with their loss of hearing, or who have not fully admitted this to themselves, mistakenly believe that *they hear all they need to hear*. The truth is, *they only hear what their hearing capacity permits*. The illusion to oneself is two-fold: you not only fail to get important information but you may not even know it; the illusion to others is that they believe communication has occurred when in fact it hasn't.

Exercise #1

Here's a little exercise I devised to help my patients quickly grasp how they're dealing with their hearing loss. Divide the top of a blank sheet of paper into three sections: on the left, title it "Situations;" in the middle "Expectations;" and on the right, title it "Actual Performance."

List three situations or environments where you expect to hear regardless of whether or not you actually can. Your task is to rate the three items under the "Expectations" and "Actual Performance" columns by selecting one of the following ratings:

NEVER - RARELY - SOMETIMES - OFTEN - ALWAYS

After you've completed this, take another piece of paper and list the same three situations, then have your spouse or someone close to you complete how they think your expectations and actual performance pan out. This makes for good and healthy discussion, and for an excellent comparison. The more truthful you are with yourself, the more you'll gain from these insights.

The Interpretation

If you've rated everything in the exercise the same for all situations, either you're an amazingly well-adjusted person with hearing loss, or you're kidding yourself. It's unlikely that all hearing situations on your list will be evaluated equally even if you are well-adjusted. So, take a closer look at your list. Bear in mind that people with normal hearing will rate the situations of expectations and performance differently because of their varying listening conditions. The difference indicates the magnitude of the problem; the greater the difference, the greater the problem. For many people with loss of hearing, it's typical to have expectations higher than performance levels. As a result, reactions to environmental situations which prove difficult can lead to the emotions discussed earlier.

The Shift to Healing

Any problem can have at least two solutions which bring about healing: (1) change the situation, or (2) change how you feel, interact or react. The problem with *changing the situation*, if you're an unaided hearing impaired person, is that you could find yourself continually changing your environment and still not hearing. You may also try to change the environment to avoid an unpleasant experience but it doesn't necessarily help you hear better.

The problem with *changing how you feel* is that it's an imposing challenge. It's very difficult to transform anger into love; frustration into understanding; or embarrassment into delight. Surely, it would seem that it doesn't happen quickly if at all. But I can tell you that I've seen it happen. When patients move past whatever has been holding them back from hearing aids, and they finally put them on, not only has a change occurred but how they feel about it becomes apparent to everyone in the room.

17

The definition of **change** is "giving up something for something else." The difficulty for anyone in making changes is that it requires giving up something to which they've grown accustomed. It is less certain, less familiar and sometimes frighteningly unknown. I've always thought that there should be a course teaching students during their first year of college how to gracefully make changes in their lives. How better adjusted to life's experiences we'd all be.

Most of us find we're not skilled in making changes. It's usually something we find uncomfortable. Even good changes are known to cause stress. A move to a better house, getting a higher paying job, or even winning the lottery cause high stress. We tend to want to stick to "the familiar." Yet, going from illness to improved health necessitates change. To avoid stress, most of us tend to stick to bad situations.

Perception has everything to do with the degree of adjustment, acceptance and solutions you embrace with regard to your hearing loss. Many people with impaired hearing report they have altered their view of the world around them in an unhealthy way. People who were once soft spoken and gentle sometimes become outspoken and angry; others, who were once alive with spirit and energy, may grow pensive and withdrawn. Those close to them notice these changes and are saddened by it. If you aren't aware of such changes, if in fact they exist, it could be because they usually develop slowly over a period of years.

If you have the courage to really look at the impact hearing loss has had on your life, the following exercise will put the truth squarely before you. After you do the exercise, read the same list to someone who knows you well (your spouse, a grown child or a close friend) and ask this person to respond *how they think you answered*, and whether or not it's true.

Exercise #2

If the statements feel mostly accurate, write True; if they feel mostly inaccurate, write False:

1) _____ I don't hear well because other people mumble, don't enunciate clearly enough, or talk too softly for me to hear.

2) _____ Since I've had this hearing loss, I can't do all the things I'd like to do.

3) _____ People don't dare make jokes about my hearing trouble in my presence.

18

4) _____ I don't mingle with as many people (old and/or new acquaintances) as I used to because I don't hear well.

5) _____ I just can't be seen wearing a hearing aid.

6) _____ If I'm left alone in a conversation, I don't understand or trust what I hear.

7) _____ I know people think I'm not as sharp as I used to be because I don't hear as well as I once did.

8) _____ If I don't want to hear what someone says the first time, I'll remain quiet; it's a waste of my time trying to hear when I can't.

9) _____ I just can't seem to assert myself the way I used to (or as others do) since I lost my ability to hear well.

10) _____ It's difficult for me to accept I actually have a hearing loss.

11) _____ I recognize that I'm the source of the problem because of my hearing loss; when I miss what somebody says to me, it's not their fault.

12) _____ Despite my hearing loss, I still do all the things I used to.

13) _____ Humorous things happen to me as a result of my not hearing well.

14) _____ In spite of my hearing loss, I'm careful not to give up any relationships I have in my life, or lose out on any potential relationships by staying home too much.

15) _____ I wouldn't think of hiding the fact that I was wearing a hearing aid.

16) _____ I feel completely at ease communicating with anyone in most environments even though I have hearing loss.

17) _____ Despite my hearing loss, other people do not think less of me than before my loss developed.

18) _____ I don't mind asking people to repeat what was said if I haven't heard it.

19) _____ As my hearing loss has developed, I've made a systematic effort to compensate for it by being more outgoing.

20) _____ It's easy for me to think of myself as having a hearing loss—it doesn't bother me.

The Interpretation

Note: Before you read the following interpretation which will give away the design of this assessment tool, be sure you have completed it fully.

Before you read this interpretation, be sure your partner has already responded to the same statements. Now then, you should know that statements 1 through 10 are the reverse of 11 through 20, respectively. For example, statement 3 is opposite to statement 13. There are two built-in veracity checks: one is that however you responded to a particular statement, if you're honest with yourself, you should have responded opposite to its corresponding statement. The other check is the way in which your partner responded.

Did you respond consistently to both sides of the statements, True on one, false on the other? Did your partner agree with you? If not, you may want to look carefully at the content of those statements. Are you denying the loss? Do you spend a lot of time with negative thinking about the loss? Are you blaming others?

Or is your outlook healthy? Do you tend to think more positively in handling your hearing loss? Do you try and find the lighter side? Are you just as engaged in life as before you developed loss of hearing?

Once you've examined the way you and your partner responded to the same statements, you may well find that you are the one person who has prevented finding your own solutions. This exercise was not an attempt to change who you are, but rather to *change and improve how you react in the world*. Don't you want better communication? Wouldn't you want to take appropriate action to help yourself? Isn't the quality of your life important enough that you care about the feelings of those close to you? Don't you want to build <u>and cross</u> that bridge to healing? With understanding and a willingness on your part to make changes, you can look forward to a whole new future.

A Personal Note

And so it goes with emotions. It can be like a summer breeze, or bull riding in a dusty pen on a 120° day. The beauty of life is that we get to choose the direction we take. We usually have choices, even when we believe we don't. If we look at hearing loss (or any problem) as an adventure—an experience to learn more about ourselves—we'll inevitably discover a brighter side to the search.

We all know that solving communication problems improves relationships. There's no mystery there. But if you think of putting your efforts toward resolution of your hearing problem as ultimately bringing that much more happiness into your life and the lives of those important to you, I think you'll readily understand and agree with the importance of resolution.

I wish to thank my wife, clinical psychologist Jo Stone-Carmen, Ph.D., whose critique of this chapter was so helpful in presenting a most sensitive topic.

CHAPTER TWO

Aging and Hearing Loss: The 50-Plus Years

James F. Maurer, Ph.D.

Dr. Maurer received his Master's Degree from Montana State University, completing doctoral studies at the University of Oregon Medical School in 1968. In 1971, he developed and directed the first mobile auditory testing and rehabilitation program in the United States for low income older persons, a program which carried on for almost two decades. He has written and co-authored seven books and many articles on hearing loss and aging. Currently, Dr. Maurer is medico-legal consultant on hearing loss associated with noise exposure, and holds an office at Portland State University in Oregon as Professor Emeritus.

You have arrived. You've earned the status in life of the "Chronologically and Biologically Elite." The survivor. Whether you're still actively working, retired and healthy, or find yourself in a protective environment because of health problems, the bottom line is that *you have survived!*

This may have mixed blessings for you, because others—precious friends and loved ones—can no longer share your experience with you. So there are moments of sadness in your achievement. Limiting health problems or fixed income may restrict some of your anticipated pleasures during later years.

Yet, you have earned the right to your own kind of happiness at this time of life. In many respects, the horizon of your life is what you make it, whether you're a new member of the club at age 50 or a seasoned veteran past the century mark. The world owes you the dignity and respect you deserve during the years ahead. Whatever life has bequeathed you in your genetic inheritance or your life experiences, good and bad, make the most of what you are. Your present physical and mental health, your financial well-being, *whatever you are* in arriving at this time in your life, take a good look in the bathroom mirror and repeat after me, "I am a survivor! I will do whatever it takes to continue to survive."

Then consider for a moment those who have supported you, not only your friends and loved ones, even your pets, past and present. They've been a support system to you. You've been special to them, and they would want you to rise above whatever limitations life has dealt.

This chapter is oriented toward people with hearing loss who have passed the fifth decade of life. It's also written for friends and family members of hearing impaired persons who have graduated from middle age and are now older husbands and wives, grandmothers and grandfathers, or singles.

What is this Thing Called "Presbycusis?"

Changes in human auditory functions due to aging begin to occur very *early* in life. You might then wonder why it's called *old age* deafness, or "presbycusis," as the word was originally coined by ancient Greeks. Diagnosticians like to diagnose, so perhaps they needed a name for this problem in their medical dictionary. More likely, their life spans being shorter in those days, people in their 40s were considered "old," with old hearing skills. Today, some examining physicians lean heavily on the patient's history. If you are an older patient and you have a hearing loss of unknown cause, the doctor is likely to diagnose the problem as presbycusis. Adding to this confusion is the fact that, while you and I may have old age *deafness*, no one ever actually became deaf from it! Even the term *hearing loss* suggests that something is terribly missing. The ears have never been the subject of much poetry anyway, as compared with the eyes, which immediately denote beauty, passion, and other emotions. Nobody ever described someone as having "bedroom ears," nor has one been portrayed as having "cauliflower" eyes.

The ears have definitely taken a beating, when it comes to anatomical derision. Small wonder that research has shown clear differences in public attitude toward people wearing hearing aids as opposed to eyeglasses. Shown pictures of the same persons with either a hearing aid or eyeglasses, viewers consistently described people wearing hearing aids as more handicapped. This stereotype is slowly changing, as ears are increasingly used for a variety of devices, from earphones pumping music or news to tiny receivers worn by broadcasters. Meanwhile, be thankful we're not living in the 13th Century when one prescription for deafness was a piece of a lion's brain stuffed in the ear with a little oil! The ears don't have it yet, but they've come a long way.

After some backsliding, most experts now agree that age-related changes that affect our hearing are in the inner ear, the auditory nerve, the brain stem, and in the auditory part of the brain. But before we collectively leap off the nearest bridge, most changes due exclusively to aging don't present a whole lot of problems. In fact, there are many older persons who can put up with a few misunderstood conversations and neither they nor their friends perceive hearing sensitivity as a problem. These folks are very fortunate.

The rest of us, myself included, not only have a touch of presbycusis, but we've picked up a few other causes of hearing loss on our trek through life, a topic you'll revisit later in this chapter and book. Meanwhile, none of us escape our later years without some loss of auditory sensitivity due to aging. We also undergo a gradual depletion of cells in the auditory processing part of our central nervous system. Once these neurons within brain stem and brain structures are depleted, they're not replaced.

Changes due to aging at this "central" level don't show up in a conventional hearing test, yet, they do account for many aging issues. There's reduced short-term memory span—"What time did you say it was?" There's lengthened reaction time to auditory signals—try keeping up with the kids in the arcade! As we age, we may experience difficulty tracking a fast-paced conversation or shifting gears to a new topic—lucky for us Walter Winchell was doing his "rapid-fire" commentary when we were kids! We might find more difficulty understanding speech—"I distinctly heard her say grushelgooch!" A recurrent problem is increased trouble understanding in background noise, particularly the "noise" of other people talking—try hearing at a political convention! And there's a greater problem paying attention—"Wake up, it's time to go home. Great sermon, wasn't it?"

Sometimes changes associated with aging can be misinterpreted as hearing impairment. An older couple came into my office for a second opinion. Urged by her husband, Mrs. Thistlebob had purchased two hearing aids, which she was wearing with some discomfort. Upon examining her I found that her hearing was normal for her age, 64 years, that she had normal speech reception and excellent discrimination of words. After testing her ability to repeat sentences presented in cafeteria noise, she was found to have a slight, but not clinically significant difficulty. In this instance, Mr. Thistlebob's perception of his wife's "hearing impairment" was incorrect.

What additional testing and discussion revealed was a significant problem with short-term memory. Her husband would ask her to bring something from another room, Mrs. Thistlebob would interrupt her activities in the kitchen to do what he asked. Then she would forget what it was that he wanted. He took this to mean that she didn't hear him, which was not so. She had simply forgotten.

Psychologists have known for years that aging affects our ability to recall things in the immediate past more than our ability to remember the distant past. Does it mean we're less intelligent as we age? No. Does it mean we're more likely to forget someone's name after just being introduced than a playmate's name recalled from childhood? Yes. Is this a NEW PROBLEM for us? No. We've forgotten things stored in short-term memory all our lives because we were distracted or focused on something else, or simply forgot. This is not "new" behavior. It's just that as we grow older, it increases in frequency. Our short-term memory "cup" runneth over more often.

Living with Loss of Hearing

Even a slight hearing impairment during this time of life may occasionally affect our ability to understand others. Since the voices of people with whom we talk vary in those characteristics that contribute to understanding, we misinterpret some individuals more than others. Voices differ in pitch, loudness, and quality, all of which can be manifested in the clarity of the speaker's voice. The actual words spoken are clearer for some individuals than others; that is, the clearer speaking person utters words that are more precisely formed, or articulated. The rate or speed of words spoken also affects our ability to understand. Messages spoken rapidly challenge our comprehension during our aging years.

Obviously, teenagers can keep up with the accelerated speech of their age group. But many of us can't keep up with them. We simply have to ask them to speak more slowly. I recall two elderly farmers sitting in a barbershop waiting for a haircut and watching the overhead television news.

"He runs all his words together," one commented. "What's he talking about?"

"He don't say," said the other. "He's not talking to us!"

Newscaster "hype" has turned to "hyper" for many of us who remember all too well the resonant and clear voices of the golden age of radio. However, there are radio and television stations which still endorse clear and reasonably paced communication. Usually, public broadcasting stations present the most understandable programming. Since some voices are clearer than others, shop around the networks for better listening experiences.

Visual cues, seeing the speaker as she or he is communicating, contribute to our getting the message. Environmental constraints on speech understanding differ considerably. Some places are virtual Towers of Babel, where sentences spoken reverberate from bare walls and floors and are lost in noise. Other rooms contain carpets and drapes and noise interference is minimized.

Places where older people congregate should be stellar listening environments. Unfortunately, this is not always the case. I recall visiting a dozen or more senior adult centers, noting the fact that while most were clean and pleasant, many were located in high noise areas and few attempts had been made to reduce interior noise. One center was actually located under a roller skating rink!

If you're reading this because you have an older parent or grandparent with hearing problems, keep in mind that it's much easier to converse with them in a quiet, carpeted room. Make sure there's good lighting and try to maintain a speaking distance of less than 9 feet. You'll be pleasantly surprised at how much easier conversation is.

It would appear that many factors interact with our loss of hearing sensitivity. Some are controllable, others are not. However, difficulty understanding speech is only one aspect of a hearing loss. To a greater or lesser extent, we monitor the world around us. Our hearing sense, as well as our vision, keep tabs on what is happening in our space. There's comfort in the constant monitoring of sounds and sights in our environment. There's a sense of belonging.

A mild hearing loss can affect how we feel. As one 56-year-old woman described to me before she began wearing hearing aids, "Not being able to hear little background sounds was like an experience I once had, sitting in an empty movie theater. I was trying to focus on the film when I realized the usual commotion of shuffling feet, popcorn crunching, hushed conversations and other sounds... were completely missing. I began to feel anxious. It was as if I were the last person alive on this planet. I got up and left the theater."

Like brush strokes on a canvas, the myriad of small sounds that we're so accustomed to hearing, tell us we are a part of reality. They also contribute to our sense of security. Detection of some warning signals may be challenging for our hearing loss, sounds such as footsteps on carpet, tires on soft snow, "fire burning in the next room," as one hapless 77-year-old apartment dweller recounted to me.

Hearing loss dampens the enjoyment of some activities that gave us pleasure in the past: public movies, music, church services, watching television, eating out, having a drink in places with background noise, talking to others on the telephone. Even a mild hearing loss can reduce life satisfaction for some things we once took for granted.

An elderly woman returned to the Audiology Clinic after a trial period of wearing hearing aids. "How did you like your new amplification?" I inquired.

"I was disgusted!" she replied. "I scrubbed my kitchen floor as soon as my friend left. Then, seeing the puzzled expression on my face," she explained, "I could hear dirt gritting under my slippers! I wonder how long it's been there?"

The specific problems that we hearing impaired older persons may experience depend on our lifestyle, the support system of friends and relatives near us, our attitudes and tolerance toward communication breakdowns, and whether we have successfully pursued professional help.

Loss of Hearing Due to Non-Aging Factors

Although we may not have significant changes in our auditory thresholds due to growing older, our loss can be compounded by other events or agents that damage our hearing mechanisms from infancy onward. A few of these include noise exposure, disease, ear infections, high fevers, head injury, toxic exposure, blood supply deficiency, and various forms of genetic deafness.

Some of these causes are preventable, such as further damaging our ears from noise exposure. Some are not, such as familial or genetic loss of hearing, although microbiologists are very close to a solution to even this problem. In any case, it's rare to find a hearing loss that is due entirely to aging, especially among men. Noise exposure is a most common cause of reduced hearing sensitivity, and because many of us pursue noisy hobbies in later years, the topic bears further discussion.

While the Occupational Safety and Health Administration (OSHA) has required noisy industries to provide ear protection since 1970, this partial solution came too late for many who are now retirement age. We live in an industrialized society where noise is seemingly omnipresent. We were endowed with eyelids to keep out most light while sleeping but no "earlids" to suppress background sounds of traffic, air conditioners, furnaces, and a host of other noise sources that are pervasive in our homes. In fact, we are indeed fortunate if we can sit quietly in the living room, close our eyes, and hear nothing.

Recreational noise has actually increased over the years with the introduction of jet sleds, all-terrain vehicles, high volume music in unwelcome places, such as shopping malls, and other experiences that relentlessly tax the sensitive structures of our inner ears. Other people's noises from automobile boom boxes, the neighborhood chain sawyer, the constant high-level drone inside some passenger planes, or 50-plus years of Fourths of July, all have a cumulative effect on our hearing. Shooting high-powered rifles, magnum pistols and shotguns is a very efficient way to lose decibels of hearing as well.

Women who are homemakers are not immune to this onslaught. Some years ago we did a sound level survey door-to-door, interviewing women and measuring the intensity of home appliances to which they were regularly exposed. Guess what took First Place honors? The loudest ruckus of the week? A vacuum cleaner generated a whopping 104 decibels at one lady's ear. That's about 20 decibels more intense than a human shout! In fact, by OSHA standards, she was running the risk of permanent hearing damage by operating that machine more than one hour a day.

Hearing loss due to age and noise are accumulative. They're not medically correctable. We can't turn the clock back and start wearing ear protectors at an earlier age, but there's something to be said for protecting what hearing we have left.

I carry an inexpensive pair of foam earplugs for use on long airplane trips and other situations where noise exposures may be loud or lengthy. In that vein, I find it interesting, having provided hearing assessments on a number of rock musicians back in the early 1970s, that many were requesting advice on hearing protectors. More recently, some now seek advice on hearing aids. I wonder about the hearing sensitivity of their audiences, the baby boomers, who within the next five years will begin joining our aging population. Thomas Edison once remarked that if we keep on inventing noisy gadgets, by the year 2000 we'll all be deaf. Having said that he continued to invent noisy gadgets.

Discovering Your Hearing Difficulty

Next time you're driving down a straight stretch on the freeway and notice that the vehicle in front of you has its turn indicator blinking incessantly, know the odds are very good that the driver has a hearing loss. And he doesn't have to be part of the aging population. The point this makes is that discovering a problem in others is often easier than in ourselves.

One very perceptive woman told me that she discovered her hearing loss when she was dining out and chatting with a companion. She noticed that she invariably stopped chewing when the other person was talking. She reasoned that the chewing noise was resonating in her head, interfering with her ability to understand; therefore, she must be experiencing reduced hearing as well, since this had never occurred before! We had to laugh at her self-assessment and decided to call it Marge's Chewing Test for Hearing Impairment.

A priest confided in me that he discovered his problem during confessions. He found himself straining to hear and missing information from soft-speaking parishioners in the booth. I was surprised to discover that his loss was not sufficient to constitute an impairment, according to the American Medical Association's guidelines; however, he did have a handicap! Later, he reported considerable relief while wearing a small canal hearing aid which he used only in the confessional booth.

A light aircraft pilot, age 61, with whom I have made several hops to various places, told me that he first noticed his hearing difficulty in court. He had been a district judge most of his later life and was now noticing problems with soft, female voices. One woman lawyer especially caused him consternation, having continually to ask her to repeat.

OSHA mandates an annual hearing test for workers exposed to potentially harmful noise. Many employees first discover that they have a loss of hearing sensitivity at the time of this test. It behooves those of us older persons who pursue noisy avocational activities in retirement (such as shop work, shooting, or running the lawn tractor over the back forty), not only to wear ear protectors but have our hearing checked on an annual basis. Get a copy of your hearing test (audiogram), so you can go home and compare it with last year's test. It's called peace of mind.

Making Adjustments to our Hearing Loss

There is diversity in how we cope with growing older. These differences are not brought on by aging. They are ways that have contributed to our uniqueness as individuals throughout our lives. Coping with a hearing loss during later years does not make us all the same either. We react in individual ways that we have always tended to react, for the primary purpose of reducing stress and solving our problems. These patterns of behavior may not always achieve conscious awareness.

Do you remember when someone first called you "Sir" or "Madame"? Did you experience a momentary flicker of surprise, an evaporating thought that you somehow must be different from that moment on? It was as if you had suddenly arrived on some plateau in life from which there was no return.

Interestingly, our arrival may have more to do with our biological age (how old we look) than our chronological age (how many birthdays we've celebrated). Some of us look our age, some of us don't. Realization of our hearing difficulties can be like that, when someone younger gives us the bad news, "Dad, you've got to do something about your hearing!" We are different from that moment on. However, for many of us there's no sudden realization. Since our loss of hearing sensitivity is gradual, it may take us a long time to recognize that we're having increasing difficulty associated with the loss.

An older couple living in a town house called this to my attention. "We used to hear the clock ticking," he said.

"What concerns me," she added, "is that we don't hear the gas jet in the fireplace anymore."

It's also interesting that some rather important sounds in our lives disappear without a whimper. Mr. Jenkins, age 74, insisted that his new hearing aid had a strange noise in it. He kept cocking his head and saying, "There it is again." Then he handed the aid to me. I listened to the instrument and shook my head. "I don't hear any noise, except normal background sounds."

Mr. Jenkins put the aid back in his ear, listening. "There it is...the noise!" After some ado, his face lit up. He realized he was hearing his own breathing!

Hearing old sounds again is like visiting old friends. It can be a positive experience. Some of us don't accept our difficulties so readily. We may in fact totally or partially deny that our problem exists. Denial has to be a cardinal quandary for the specialist trying to rehabilitate some folks. Typical "denial" statements are sometimes plausible and sometimes not. For example, "I'm sorry, I wasn't paying attention," or, "You're mumbling again," may be ways of concealing that we have hearing difficulties. These diversionary statements should not be judged. They're simply learned methods of protecting ourselves and reducing the stress of facing a hearing problem.

John was a 70-year-old longshoreman who came to my office announcing that his doctor told him he had the arteries of a 30-year-old. He flexed his triceps and asked me to feel them. "Hard as steel," I responded, knowing what was coming next.

"Doc," he shouted, "I don't have any trouble hearing. I don't know why they sent me here. I can hear a pin drop."

But he couldn't. In fact, he couldn't hear a brick drop. Not only that, he couldn't understand conversational level speech. And ability to hear in noise? Forget it!

I always feel saddened by such patients. They want to stay young. They want to have youthful hearing skills. They don't want to wear hearing aids because they see them as another indication that their bodies are growing older. Here was a macho man swimming against the current of aging. And who can blame him?

One of the reasons why denial takes place is manifested by the configuration of the hearing loss. When we look at our audiogram (the hearing test), most of us see a hearing sensitivity curve that drops off, getting poorer, in the high frequencies. We may still hear low-pitched sounds very well, but we don't hear higher-pitched sounds. Thus, telling this person, "You're not hearing!" is not entirely true. Some sounds may be heard quite well. Others may not be heard at all. Nevertheless, our ever-active brain fills in the blanks, sometimes correctly, sometimes not.

Grandpa and his grandson Joey were painting the shed. Joey said, "Gramps, let's go get some **thinner**."

Grandpa laughed and shook his head incredulously. "**Dinner?** Why son, we just had lunch!"

This illustrates the difference between <u>hearing</u> and <u>understanding</u>. Joey's grandfather *thought* he heard the message. In fact, he correctly heard five out of six words spoken by his grandson. But he didn't hear one critical consonant, the soft /th/ sound, so his brain tried to fill in the blank. This small misperception changed the entire meaning of his grandson's request. When this starts happening to us frequently in conversations with others, perhaps we're overdue in asking for help!

Many of us endure the typical high frequency hearing loss that Grandpa experiences. Such a loss allows us to hear the louder "vowelized" speech sounds, as in the word /I/, but we have trouble with the softer consonant sounds in words such as **th**igh. These voiceless consonant sounds, speech sounds like /f/ in "fish," /s/ in "see" contribute <u>most</u> to our ability to understand human communication. Not hearing them because they're made even softer by our hearing loss creates errors for us in interpreting messages. So our denial may surface simply because we hear *some* sounds well and can therefore reject the thought that we have much difficulty hearing others.

The high frequency loss may create a quandary for us when we *see* a bird singing, but don't *hear* his song, or when someone draws our attention to the chirping of crickets, the whisper of wind in the trees, or the swishing of clothing. Missing a sound also can be serious.

Mrs. Wolford described the experience of an injurious accident caused by her impairment. "I was walking through the park, admiring the autumn colors all around me on a beautiful September day. Suddenly, a speeding bicycle was at my elbow. I sidestepped, thinking to avoid a collision, but instead I fell painfully to the sidewalk. The boy stopped, helped me up, and apologized for frightening me. The truth is it was not his fault. There was no need for my sudden reaction. I should have heard his bicycle coasting through the leaves."

We can make errors in interpreting what someone is saying or even doing, sometimes with embarrassing or even painful consequences. If this doesn't happen very often, it's easier to deny that it happens at all.

While high frequency hearing loss during later years is characterized by the situations just described, many other individuals have reduced sensitivity across the frequency spectrum. Those of us who do have difficulty hearing <u>both</u> high- and low-pitched speech sounds experience greater deprivation. If such a loss is mild, we may not hear any words spoken in quiet conversation. When the loss is severe, we may not perceive conversational level speech at all. Hearing the telephone or the doorbell ringing may be difficult if we are not positioned close enough to these sounds. Most people around us have to raise their voices so that we may hear. When we experience this kind of auditory dysfunction, we know we need help. And the sooner the better.

I used to routinely advise people with hearing aids to take them off before going to bed. One 82-year-old woman was offended by that statement as a cardinal rule. "I've slept on my left side and worn one hearing aid in my right ear for over 10 years," she admonished. "Who knows who might be knocking on my door in the middle of the night? Or what if the phone rings? I might miss something!"

A few individuals take immediate and aggressive action to

counteract a recently discovered hearing difficulty. One gentleman bounced into my office like a bandy rooster one morning, gesturing wildly and shouting, "How do I get some hearing aids!"

When I asked him why he thought he needed them, he said that he no longer could understand his patent attorneys at monthly board meetings. "I have to depend on what they say. Trouble is, they mumble separately. If they mumbled collectively," he quipped, "I think I'd understand what they were talking about." He wanted a quick solution, and he wasn't about to let a hearing impairment stand in his way. This was a man who was used to making adjustments. He was 82 years old. Did I say "old?" I mean *young!*

Others of us refuse to accept our impairments as we do our chronological age, by ignoring senior citizen discounts in restaurants and malls, because of the embarrassment in admitting the truth. A few even disassociate from people their own age. Similarly, we may ignore the pleas of others by not appearing in clinics willingly. Often, our late appearance is a begrudging one, something we're doing for "them," but not for ourselves. Some even deny that they want to hear. "Look, I can hear most things around me," a 57-year-old attorney said, folding his arms. "There's a whole lot going on out there that I don't want to hear. I do just fine." His wife sat quietly in the corner, looking very tired.

Often, our reluctance to seek help presents a barrier to those attempting to talk with us. If straining to hear is fatiguing, imagine what it must be like for another person who has to keep repeating all day.

The denial of aging is often projected as a stigma against hearing aids which are for "older" persons. This can become an attitudinal disclaimer that hearing difficulty is not an important part of our lives. A glass of water won't suffice when we're thirsting for the Fountain of Youth. Some of us even engineer our lives to convince ourselves that we hear normally. We simply minimize our exposure to situations where the hearing deficit compromises our enjoyment of life!

I asked a woman in her late fifties, "What things did you do 10 years ago that gave you a lot of satisfaction?"

She responded, "Let's see, I was very active in the church. I really enjoyed that. I taught Sunday School. I went to a symphony about once a month. Oh, and bridge club. That meant a lot to me 10 years ago."

"Are you still enjoying these activities?"

She was quiet for a moment. "Well no, not really," she shrugged. "It became too much work teaching those children, and too much fussing to get ready for the symphony. I moved onto other things, I guess."

As we talked on, it became clear that she had sacrificed part of her life satisfaction because of increasing hearing difficulties. She had carefully limited her activities so that the impairment wouldn't affect her life. And she had accomplished this without ever admitting that the cause of her withdrawal was her inability to hear. Fortunately, this woman turned out to be an excellent candidate for aural rehabilitation, where she was involved in group counseling. Once she could identify with other women in the group who had similar problems, her self-esteem increased and she began to move out of her self-imposed isolation.

Because there are situations where we honestly feel we can hear normally, in front of a blasting television, for example, it becomes easy to blame others for our social inadequacy. In the hearing health care field, many of us have heard the following during an interview with an older couple.

"**He** doesn't hear what I'm saying."

"**She** doesn't speak up!"

When you think about it, we all project our problems onto other people or other things at some point in our lives. How many times have we heard statements like, "I know where I got this miserable cold—that sneezing kid in the shopping mall," or, "You forgot to remind me that I had a meeting."

There's nothing unique about a hearing impaired person projecting his or her problem. We all need a scapegoat at times, in order to reduce our stress. Similarly, we may find withdrawal appropriate for some situations, such as a frustrating conversation in a noisy room. These ways of avoiding or escaping from stress, denying the problem, compensating for it, projecting it, withdrawing from it actually make us feel better when our backs are against the wall. They help us maintain a positive self-image, which takes a beating when we can't hear well. But if carried too far, these bailout behaviors can interfere with getting help and reduce our life satisfaction.

Compromising our lives in order to convince ourselves that we hear normally is an all-too-common experience among those of us with impairments. Like the woman described earlier, curtailing formerly enjoyed activities can seriously reduce enjoyment of life! If you find you're no longer showing up at holiday parties, club activities, homes of friends or other previously reinforcing events, take a look in that mirror again. Maybe it's time to seek professional help.

What's also missing here is social responsibility. We hearing impaired people owe others the right to conversations that are free of frustration. We owe our friends freedom from continually having to repeat conversations. We owe them an honest appraisal of our hearing difficulties.

What is not realized by many of us is that once we can hear better, we may discover a rebirth of more youthful participation in social activities. We become better social companions. As one wife exclaimed, "When he puts those hearing aids on, he's more like himself."

Retiring Comfortably with a Hearing Loss

It's interesting to talk to people with auditory problems who have recently retired. Some experience a sudden loss of power, the ingratiating experience of sliding backwards down the slope that leads to nonperson status in the eyes of once admiring co-workers. Normal hearing people may experience the same thing. This was the feeling that a recently retired physician related to me. His repeated returns to his beloved medical school, where he had held an office for more than 30 years, were met with disengaging smiles and chafing comments like, "What are YOU doing back here?" He began questioning whether a prejudice was operating because of his new hearing aids, his whiter-than- others' hair, and the fact that he was retired. Ultimately, he felt that his once respected opinion no longer mattered, and with some reluctance, he ended his visits.

Some years later after my own retirement, he called me. "You know," he said, "if you ever write another book or have to counsel a lonely retiree, you might remember this piece of advice: if you live alone and your world is passing you by, be grateful for what you have left. Then, make yourself important to someone. You'll be pleasantly surprised how important you become to yourself."

He was embarking on his third trip to China to help children with birth defects. He had decided that nothing could get in the way of his need to help others, neither hearing aids, aging body, nor unresponsive colleagues.

We are a diverse population, we older persons. Some of us cross over to retirement more slowly, tenaciously clinging to our previous

34

roles in life through occasional work or social and service activities. We may express joy at having left our working selves behind. We network with friends seeking a newfound freedom, finding companionship in the excitement of long awaited travel, new recreational activities, educational pursuits, or greater involvement in hobbies. Some of us don't retire at all.

Hearing loss does not respect our differences. We find individuals with auditory difficulties in all lifestyles. What's important is that we don't let this problem curtail our pleasures in life. A pharmacist friend who had been a trap shooter since boyhood was left with a significant high frequency hearing impairment in both ears. He wears two hearing aids now in retirement, and when I visit his home I always take a handful of earplugs. He constructed a woodworking shop in his garage and now creates quality furniture both as a hobby and to supplement his pension.

He and his wife are very happy in retirement, and I was prompted to ask him, "If you had it to do over, would you give up 30 years of shooting?"

"No, I wouldn't give that up. Nor these either," he grinned, pointing to his hearing aids.

Enjoyment is found in a quiescent lifestyle for many of us. Our activities may be limited to television viewing, reading, eating, sleeping, and occasionally making visits to friends, relatives, church, and senior adult centers. We find pleasure where we can and enjoy predictability in our lives.

One such individual, age 72, has neuropathy in his hands. Because of this lack of feeling, he can no longer operate his hearing aid. He has been perfectly content with his adjustment to his hearing impairment because his lifestyle does not involve a great number of social activities. He's an avid sports fan, and enjoys watching these contests vicariously. One of his concessions to his hearing difficulty is a pair of earphones connected to an infrared television amplifying system. This "assistive listening device" is easy to manipulate. It allows him to turn up baseball games as loud as he wants without interfering with adjoining apartment tenants. He also has a telephone amplifier. Such devices, described in Chapter 13, are very useful in supplementing or substituting for traditional hearing aids.

Regaining life satisfaction may mean letting go of some of our former attitudes about aging and hearing loss and beginning to accept the realities of a new emerging self. It helps to take stock of all the positive attributes in our lives. There are people who like us for who we are, wrinkles be damned. They could care less about our need for prosthetic devices. They care about us. They accept our baggage. In fact, it becomes so much a part of us that the people we care about don't even see it anymore.

It also helps to look around at the place where we spend most of our waking hours. What are the positive attributes in our home environment? What things produce pleasure for us? If we close our eyes, how many of these things would no longer be pleasurable, such as a picture that is dear to us or a good book? If we could close our ears and hear nothing, what things of enjoyment would be missed?

Now take inventory of positive activities outside the home, things we like to do with our time. This could include hobbies, meetings, entertainment, and activities that are more physical, such as walking, fishing, travel, golf. If we apply the same limitations to our activities, in turn, closing our eyes and ears, what would the effect be? What enjoyable activities would we have to give up?

What we discover from this simple exercise is that first, there are many positive things operating in each of our lives. Getting older is not a virus that takes away all our satisfaction with life. Second, recounting our pleasures with two of our senses "closed" eliminates many positive aspects of our lives that we would not give up willingly.

Now hang on to that thought, because not giving up is exactly the attitude that must persist if we are to realize our most positive potential in spite of our hearing loss. This means accepting ourselves wearing devices that will open up a part of the world's pleasures which would otherwise be forsaken. It means accepting our new selves.

Interestingly, the world will accommodate our new self-image, and we can now move forward with our lives. People began to like us better because we are *real* in projecting who we are, and we're happier for that experience. Popeye probably said it best, "I am what I am, and that's what I am!" Did he wear hearing aids? You mean you didn't notice?

Hearing aids are compensatory mechanisms. In wearing them we are making a statement to ourselves that an impairment is not an acceptable alternative, especially when it can be helped. We consciously or unconsciously make other adjustments as well during the aging process. Our eyes admit less light than in former years, so we try to adjust our reading habits accordingly, or reduce some activities such as night driving. Ability to understand conversations in background noise becomes diminished, so we try to avoid the incompatible combination of noisy places and conversations. We find quieter places to converse. Knowledge of reduced physical stability makes us move more cautiously in risky situations where we might fall, such as taking a shower, getting into the bathtub, climbing a ladder. We discover that sudden movements can produce dizziness or unsteadiness, so we avoid quick changes in position. Diets may change to cope with the most prevalent disorder after age 45— vascular disease. We find ourselves getting less sleep at night because of awakenings, and may discover a decrease in the quality of sleep. So we may compensate with naps. And the list goes on.

Compensating for perceived changes is a healthy, friendly way of insuring survival. It is taking charge of one's life. It's making a positive statement about the aging years! Like the old adage that a graying dowager told me years ago, "There may be snow on the roof, but there's fire in the furnace!" And stoking that furnace, managing one's life experiences, reducing the impact of a hearing difficulty by acknowledging the problem to others, getting professional help, and arranging our living places so we can hear better, are giant steps in the right direction.

Taking Charge of the Environment

Arranging where we reside, eat, work, play or pray means getting closer to the source of sound, for example, television, stereo, church pew, or the waitress in a cafe. What we're accomplishing by favorably positioning ourselves in living situations is improvement in understanding communication. The greater the distance we are from the sound source, the more distortion we'll experience, whether we realize it or not. Besides, there are visual cues: facial expressions, mouth movements, gestures, and body language. These nuances of visual communication may not be visible from a distance but do actually clarify the message up close. Prove it to yourself. Stand six feet or so from an older friend. Tell this person, "I want you to spell this word." Now cover your face with a large manilla envelope or something and at normal loudness say the word, "fin." If the person gets it right, which is highly unlikely, try it with someone else. If the wrong word is spelled, such as "pin" or "sin," immediately uncover your face and say "fin" again. The friend should get it correct with visual cues. This makes a point, whether you actually do it or not.

Everyone lip-reads to a certain extent, but most people don't realize the importance in "seeing" speech.

Stage-managing our lives also means getting away from distracting or overpowering noise or loud music. One may enjoy the power of organ music and sit close to it in a place of worship, but at what cost to hearing the message? Think of places in your life where it's difficult to hear: driving or riding in an automobile, sitting in the breakfast nook adjacent to the humming of appliances, standing at the cash register in a busy restaurant, or before the agent in a bus terminal. Make a list of these noisy places in your life and then think, **quiet**! Ask, "How can I adjust my daily living to make hearing easier?" For example, some cars are quieter than others. Look in consumer magazines, where advice is published on "quieter" interiors of automobiles. Your spouse or friend riding co-pilot will be grateful. But so will you.

Oh, how tough it is for many of us to say: "I have a hearing problem!" Especially to strangers and new acquaintances. I have a friend who I meet for lunch periodically. He wears two hearing aids that aren't particularly visible, since they're skin-tone in color and recessed somewhat in his ear canals. What he does is rather interesting. He always takes charge of the situation by looking at the waitress in a friendly way and asking her a neutral question, such as, "How long have you worked here?" When she responds, he smiles and nods his head. But if he has difficulty understanding her, he gently grasps her sleeve or wrist and pulls her toward him, sometimes adding, "There, I can hear you better now." Frankly, when I first saw him doing this, I had visions of testifying on his character in a harassment suit. But for him, it works. (Okay, except once, when the waitress allowed him to pull her closer to the booth. But then, upon noticing his hearing aids, she bellowed her answer in a voice so loud it lifted both of us off our chairs!)

Adaptation to a gradual loss of sensitivity takes place slowly. It's manifested by more subtle ways of compensating for diminishing hearing, often unconscious ways, that sometimes signal to others the presence of our reduced auditory comprehension. These behaviors may happen before the person with the hearing loss is even aware of it. If we could see a video tape of ourselves during episodes of hearing difficulty, we would be surprised at the subtle cues that may not escape notice by others. Like peacocks, we stretch our heads forward to hear a friend talking in the background noise of a group. Some frown incessantly, straining to understand what someone is saying. We may establish intense eye contact with the speaker. We find ourselves asking people to repeat, often unconsciously and often a number of times in a single conversation. A few of us even cup one hand behind an ear to increase the sound a few decibels. Or giving up on the situation, we simply nod in agreement without really understanding the message. Most of these behaviors we've exhibited since childhood, but what we don't realize is they're increasing in frequency.

Helping Yourself to Hear Again

Art Carney, famed co-comedian on, "The Honeymooners," with Jackie Gleason, once walked out on the stage to perform, only to discover that his hearing aid battery was dead. He knew he could neither hear well nor react to his cues, so he openly admitted his problem to the audience and related the following story which has been bantered around at cocktail parties ever since. Maybe you haven't heard it. Carney said that a friend raved about his new hearing aid. Listening to music was wonderful. He could hear sounds that he hadn't heard since childhood. He could even hear conversations spoken in noise with this new hearing aid!

"What kind is it?" Carney asked him.

"Three o'clock," his friend replied.

Hearing appliances have been the brunt of jokes since they first appeared on the market. Older persons may remember the mastodons sold to their parents or grandparents—bulky, unappealing devices that clearly made a statement that the wearer was "deaf" and possibly a little strange, as well.

We live in an extended past, all of us. While the mastodon aid is now buried in history, many individuals continue to be reluctant to accept hearing instruments. The manufacturers know this and hearing aids have become smaller and smaller, presumably to hide the "defect." Hearing aids have not become as fashionable as eyeglasses, despite the fact that we can be helped by tiny ear devices which offer considerably less visibility.

Even the label of "deafness" over more acceptable terms, such as "nearsighted" or "farsighted," seems to be a more global pronouncement. I recall seeing a sign on an old wooden building outside Salem, Oregon that advertised, "Coffins and Hearing Aids." Unfortunately, if I noticed that sign so did thousands of others. I wonder how many older persons lived on without doing anything about their hearing problem because of the thoughtless association of those two words.

Our reluctance to get help actually may stem from any of several factors, which surfaced in a survey we once conducted among several thousand older persons. Vanity (how we perceive our appearance) was the most prevalent reason. Most of us find wearing eyeglasses more fashionable than hearing aids. Perceived geographic isolation from clinics providing hearing instruments ranked high on the survey, as well as lack of mobility. Older folks tend to view other health problems as more serious than their hearing impairment. My opinion to those in my age group who also have hearing difficulties is that there are ample reasons for finding out what gains these instruments can offer. We may lose more by not trying them.

Helping a Loved One in a Restricted Environment

If you know someone in a nursing home is benefiting from a hearing aid or two, keep tabs on their ability to use them. Does this person have the skills and dexterity to put the instruments in the ear, turn them up, and remove them before going to bed? Can the individual change the batteries when appropriate? Is the family physician checking to see that the ear canals are free of wax build-up? Does the nursing staff complain of hearing aid whistling? This "feedback" can be caused by earwax. Is someone remembering to open up the battery doors at night, saving on battery life during sleeping hours?

And while we're at it, is anybody cleaning this person's glasses once in a while? Remember, visual skills also help the hearing impaired person. If your loved one can no longer manage the prosthetic devices, ask who in the nursing staff is responsible. In many cases I've witnessed, the primary person who cares and oversees the maintenance of your loved one's prosthetic devices is you!

Strange things happen to hearing aids in nursing homes. They can be stolen, substituted for someone else's instrument down the hall, uncomfortably stuck in the wrong ear, chewed on or digested by someone's visiting dog or cat, dropped in the toilet, plugged with wax, sentenced to lifetime solitary confinement in a dresser drawer, stepped on by a 250-pound attendant, or awaiting invitation under the bed to the fraternal order of dust bunnies.

If the instrument seems to be helping the older person only by making him or her more alert, take this as a positive sign and reward the use of hearing aids. If you make a visit and find it's not being worn, check to make sure the aids are working. It's wise of you to participate in getting the hearing aids in the ears during your visit. Chances are your warm gestures of touching, smiling, talking and caring will have positive consequences on this special person. And on you, as well.

You may be reading this book to find out what you can do for a loved one who sadly can no longer understand the printed word, cannot write effectively, or may be wandering in that personal void associated with severe mental deterioration. Unfortunately, the lower the level of intellectual functioning, the poorer the prognosis for gaining much benefit from amplification. But check first to see if increasing the volume of the soothing sound of your voice seems to create a pleasant experience, or even an increase in understanding.

I took some graduate students to a nursing home to do hearing testing on some residents. One gentleman who we saw sat very quietly in a corner of the hallway not socializing with anyone. He just looked emptily at the opposite wall. One of the staff told us he had been diagnosed aphasic, which is lack of speech understanding and expression due to brain damage. We had brought with us a powerful body hearing aid with a big red volume control. We placed it in a harness on his body, hooked his right ear up to it, and slowly began turning up the volume. His mouth opened slightly, his head turned toward us, and as we watched, a wisp of a smile turned into a full-fledged grin. One student tried to subdue her excitement and quietly asked, "Can you hear me, Mr. Jackson?"

He looked at her, eyes glistening, and managed a, "Yuh...Yes!" A few weeks later, after we had showed him how to use the aid and charge the battery each night, I returned to see how he was doing. I found him sitting on the sun porch, holding hands with an elderly woman, talking quietly. The big box with the red volume control still hung on his chest.

A Look to the Future

Important advances in hearing aids and in genetic engineering have been made since this aid with the red knob was constructed. Before we acquiesce to the ticking of genetic alarm clocks slowly ringing down the curtain on our lives, there's much to be optimistic about. Microbiologists have recently succeeded in doubling life expectancy. Although it was only a lowly worm, it's a beginning! They have a big reason to work hard on this. After all, they're aging too! Also, we may yet live to see some forms of hereditary deafness denied access to our genetic makeup.

Similarly, electronic advances in digital processing are beginning to penetrate that old amplification bugaboo, trying to understand someone talking in conversational noise. Modern hearing instruments do help. Efforts in designing programmable instruments, while still evolving, are demonstrating positive consequences for senior hearing aid users. So, for the present, we older people must sustain ourselves with the thought that while our hearing losses and aging selves cannot be miraculously restored to youthful states, forces are decidedly moving in our favor.

CHAPTER THREE

The Process of Hearing Loss

H. Gustav Mueller, Ph.D.

Dr. Mueller received his Doctorate in Audiology from the University of Denver in 1976. He has an audiology consulting practice with a home office in the mountains west of Boulder, Colorado. He has been fitting and writing about hearing aids for 25 years. Dr. Mueller is a Founder of the American Academy of Audiology and holds faculty positions with Vanderbilt University and Nova Southeastern University. He is the Contributing Editor for The Hearing Journal, has written over 100 articles, and a number of professional book chapters in the field.

My first introduction to hearing impairment came when I was a young boy growing up on a farm in North Dakota with my parents, who were in their late fifties at the time. In particular, I have a vivid memory of the summer of 1958; during the long hot days I would spend my time on an old Model D John Deere tractor, following my father on his tractor, field after field, performing a task called, "summer fallowing." Basically, this meant attacking tons of huge rag weeds with a cultivator, traditional summer work performed by my brothers 20 years before me. My mother spent her days at the farmstead, baking, keeping the creaky old farmhouse immaculately clean, and doing the farmyard chores. Late at night, after dinner (*supper* in our family), and dishes were finished, the three of us would take a few minutes and sit out on the front porch in the cool nighttime air to share the events of the day (I always had one or two good weed stories to tell).

As time would go on, the conversation between my parents would get to the part that I always found the most intriguing. It usually would go something like this.

"Herman," my Mother would say, "step on that cricket over there by you, that sound is driving me crazy!"

"What cricket?" Dad would reply. "I don't hear any cricket! I think you're hearing things!"

At this point, I would usually chime in with something like, "Dad, I don't believe you can't hear the cricket!"

This would prompt my Mom to say, "Herman, you know you really should have your hearing checked, there's a lot of things that you don't hear."

Forty years of running threshing machines and sitting on old "put-put" tractors hadn't been kind to my Dad's ears, but, as an old German farmer, he didn't believe in doctors (especially when no blood was involved), and this kind of talk from my Mom really irritated him. He always had a good comeback. "Bernice, I think it's you that has a hearing problem. How about this morning during milking. I heard the train pulling out of Ryder (a small town about three miles away), and you never heard it. How can I have a hearing problem if I hear things that you can't hear?"

This is where I became puzzled. Did he have a hearing loss or didn't he? He had been known to make up things just to get out of an uncomfortable situation, but I had confirmed the train story one day when we were outside together. On the other hand, I knew darn well he couldn't hear the crickets. I'd also noticed when we were riding in our noisy old 1946 Ford pickup, I'd always have to repeat things. He said it was my fault, of course. Something about the fact that I mumbled—maybe I did.

I soon became a teenager and decided that it wasn't "cool" to sit on the porch with my parents, but I'm guessing that the same talk about hearing challenges continued year after year. Time went on. I went off to college and in 1971 I received my Master's Degree in Audiology. Those porch-time conversations all made sense now. I learned that noise exposure can cause a permanent hearing loss, but usually only affects the high frequencies (pitches). Quite often, hearing for low frequencies remains excellent (like the rumbling of a distant train). I learned that one of the first signs of a high frequency noise-induced hearing loss is that people have trouble understanding speech when there's background noise. In one of my counseling courses, I also learned that people often deny that they have a hearing problem—they think it's a sign of getting old. It's too bad we all didn't know that back in 1958. By the way, in the spring of 1972, just before the wheat crop went in, I fit my first pair of hearing aids—to my father.

So, you now know a little bit about my father and his hearing loss. Unfortunately, even today, similar stories are told in families all over the U.S. Lets do some math. As I related to you, I can remember that he had a hearing problem as far back as 1958—I'm sure he had problems long before that. When did he receive his first hearing aids? **1972!** And only then because I pulled him into Minot State College for testing. My best guess is that for 20 years or more, my father needed hearing aids, but did not seek help. Did it cause him problems? Of course. I can remember a Christmas gathering in the late 1960s at my brother's house. In a room filled with many conversations and children playing, my father sat in a corner by himself. Family members initially had tried to include him in conversations, but gave up after awhile, as they tired of repeating everything. He had tried to keep up with the multiple conversations, but soon gave up. It was just too much work. Is it any wonder why he tried to avoid family gatherings? Would hearing aids have solved *all* the problems? Probably not. Would they have made a significant improvement? Absolutely!

If you have a hearing loss, or if a family member or acquaintance of yours has a hearing problem, there are some things that you can do to assure that the potential negative consequences of the issues surrounding it are avoided or minimized. I think you'll find that it's easier to make decisions if you have a general understanding of the problem. There are two key factors that interrelate to create a hearing loss handicap: the components of sound (especially speech sounds) and the function (or dysfunction) of the ear. With a basic understanding of these two factors, we can then talk about the tests that are used to assess hearing. But first, let's be clear about the kind of hearing loss you may have.

Types of Hearing Loss

There are three main types of hearing loss: *conductive* hearing losses are caused by an obstruction of the sound pathway into the inner ear; *sensorineural* hearing losses are caused by damage to the nerve cells located in the inner ear; and *mixed* hearing losses are combinations of both conductive and sensorineural losses. Conductive hearing losses are sometimes correctable by surgery or medicine. They may be caused by middle ear infections, wax accumulation, ruptured eardrums, or a disorder of the middle ear bones which connect the eardrum to the inner ear. Sensorineural losses, often called "nerve type," are seldom correctable and are caused by aging, loud noise exposure, infection, viruses, and genetic disorders. A person with a mixed hearing loss may be someone who has lost hearing due to exposure to loud sounds, such as gunfire, and, in addition, has wax blocking the ear canal. If you have a conductive hearing loss, you generally hear quite well when sound is made loud enough to overcome the obstruction in the sound pathway. However, if you have a sensorineural hearing loss, you may notice distortion of speech sounds even when the sounds are loud enough for you to hear. More about this later.

What Is Sound?

You've all heard the saying about a tree falling in the middle of a forest. If no one's there, does it make a sound? If sound is only defined as something we hear, then the answer would be *no*. In the physical sense, the answer would be *yes*, as all the properties of sound were present. So, remember that you can have sound without hearing, but you cannot have hearing without sound.

Vibrations

Sound is vibrations. Vibrations are caused by wave motion. The surface waves of water, and radio waves are also examples of particles set into vibration by waves. In the case of sound, it is air particles that are set into motion. Imagine sitting in your favorite chair in your living room, about 10 feet from your piano. The air molecules in that room are all packed tightly together, and are packed against your eardrum (it doesn't feel like pressure to you because there are air molecules on the other side of your eardrum to equalize the effect). Air molecules are also packed tightly around the strings of the piano. Now, someone strikes the middle-C key, the hammer strikes the string and the string begins to vibrate. Every movement of that string bumps the air molecules next to it, which in turn bump the next molecules, and within a hundredth of a second, this bumping action has made its way to the air molecules located next to your eardrum. The result: the air molecules bump against your eardrum and set it into motion and you hear the tone. In this example the process would repeat itself 256 times/second, as that is the number of vibrations of the middle-C piano string (unless your piano needs to be tuned!).

Speed of Sound

The bumping together of air molecules allows sound to travel from one place to another. This determines the velocity, or speed of sound. At sea level, sound waves travel at 1130 feet/second, which corresponds to 770 miles/hour. While in some respects this is fast, it's much slower than the speed of light, which is essentially instantaneous. This, of course, is why we can play the summertime game of "how far away is the storm," by counting the seconds between the time that we see the lightning and then hear the thunder.

Now that we understand there are these air particles bouncing all over, it's time to consider three important components of these particles: intensity, frequency, and spectrum.

Intensity

If we were to visually display sounds, we would see that different sound waves have different strengths (which can result in different loudness levels). Lets go back to our piano example. The harder someone strikes the key, the harder the hammer strikes the string, and the greater the string deviates from its resting position. The harder strike *does not* cause the string to vibrate faster (that would be frequency), it simply changes the force on the molecules next to the string, which ultimately changes the force on the molecules that are bumping (or banging) against your eardrum. When the piano string pushed the air molecules next to it, work was being done, and energy was expended. With sound, we measure this energy using the term intensity.

The Decibel

Usually, the intensity of a sound is expressed in decibels. The term originated from telephone engineers who derived the "Bel" in honor of Alexander Graham Bell, which is why the "B" is capitalized in the abbreviation "dB." (By the way, the plural of the abbreviation dB is still dB, not *dBs*.) The decibel scale is not like most other scales with which you may be familiar. The decibel is expressed as a ratio. For this reason, relatively small decibel increments can result in large changes in ratios. A 10 dB increase in intensity is a 100 times increase in the intensity ratio.

Here's an example from the field of music. If I said that at a recent rock concert, the band performed their music 10 dB louder than Barry Manilow, it wouldn't seem like a big deal. After all, it's only 10 dB. However, if I told you that the rock band's music was *100 times* louder than Mr. Manilow's, you might start thinking that the band was playing pretty darn loud!

Intensity versus Loudness

Loudness is your psychological reaction to intensity. I could play a 70 dB SPL noise to 10 different people, and they could all give me a different loudness rating. What's "comfortably loud" to one person might be "just a little too loud" to another. If you doubt this, listen in on the conversation of a married couple as they're deciding on the volume adjustment of their television set!

This is an important concept in the selection and fitting of hearing aids. You and your friend might have the exact same hearing loss, but your loudness judgments might be different for louder sounds. Hearing aids need to be adjusted for your specific loudness judgments. This is where the physical and psychological aspects of sound work together to form the right match.

Frequency

As the name suggests, frequency refers to the number of vibrations of sound that occur in one second. That is, a tone of 1000 Hz is a tone with a frequency of 1000 cycles per second. If you could somehow take your index finger and move it back and forth 100 times/second, you would actually hear a corresponding low frequency sound. You've probably seen a tuning fork at your family physician's office. These devices are used to generate frequency-specific pure tones. Indeed, when the fork is struck, the tines vibrate at a specific rate/second which corresponds to standard frequency values. The same applies to our previous example of the piano string, which was vibrating at the rate of 256 times each second—referred to as middle-C. In the past, this vibration rate was referred to as cycles per second, or cps. Today, the preferred term is Hertz, abbreviated "Hz," named in honor of Heinrich Rudolf Hertz, a German physicist.

The range of human hearing is usually considered to be between 20 and 20,000 Hertz. Not too many sounds of interest to us occur at either extreme. The range necessary for understanding speech is from about 125 to 6000 Hz. At an early age, our hearing begins to become poorer for the ultra-high frequencies (above 12,000 Hz), so it's good that most of the important speech signals are at 6000 Hz or below. The frequency range of speech does not vary too much from speaker to speaker, although you may characterize a person as having a deeper voice than another. The high frequency sounds of speech, however, are similar for all people talking. Therefore, the person with a high frequency hearing loss usually will have difficulty understanding all speakers. In particular, problems will occur when listening to women or children. This is not because the pitch is higher, but because these two groups tend to produce less high frequency energy when they speak.

The Audiogram

An audiogram is a graph used to display your hearing ability. Decibels have been converted on an audiogram (by a mathematical formula) from sound pressure levels (SPL), the levels that we hear in the real world—to hearing levels (HL), what we hear through the audiometer (equipment used to measure hearing). Therefore, on the audiometer, 0 dB does not represent the complete absence of sound, but is simply a reference level for the softest sound that the best of normal hearing people will hear 50 percent of the time.

To put the audiogram scale in perspective, average speech sounds range from around 20 to 60 dB; rustling leaves are around 20-25 dB, the roar of a jet engine would be 100 dB or more. The decibel scale on the audiogram ranges from -10 to 120 dB. Remember, the zero dB point is an average reference level for excellent hearing. If your hearing is extremely good, you might hear better than average, which would be a minus value. The normal hearing range is defined as the ability to hear all tones that are 20 dB or softer.

Because the primary purpose of the clinical hearing test is to determine your ability to hear average speech sounds, the frequencies of the clinical audiogram only address this range. Additionally, to simplify frequency selection and help us remember all the octave and half-octave values, all audiometric frequencies are even multiples of 50 Hz. For example, we use 250 rather than 256, 500 rather than 512, and so on. A routine hearing test, therefore, would include the following frequencies: 250, 500, 1000, 2000, 3000, 4000, 6000, and 8000 Hz.

So, now that you have this information for both intensity and frequency, it's time to take a look at an audiogram. Shown in Figure 3-1 is an audiogram that provides you with some examples for both frequency and intensity. The gray area, shaped like a banana, is the range for average speech (yes, even scientists call it the "speech banana"). For specific speech examples, look in the upper right portion and you will see the speech sounds of /f/, /s/, and /th/, located around the 4000-6000 range at 20 dB. In contrast, the /z/ and /v/ sounds are located around 250-500 Hz at 30 dB. We've included several environmental sounds on the audiogram too, to give a general perspective of the world around you.

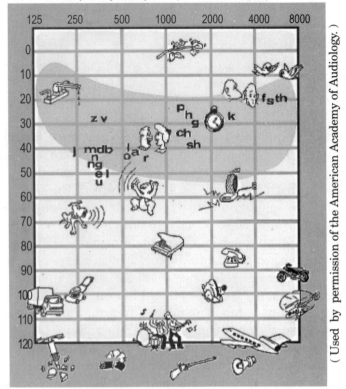

Figure 3-1: Pictorial representation of the
frequency and intensity of sounds.

Frequency versus Pitch

Just as loudness is the psychological correlate to intensity, pitch is the psychological correlate to frequency. Not all of us would judge a 1000 Hz signal as having the same pitch. Also, some people are better than others at differentiating one pitch from another. When fitting hearing aids, your provider will use your judgments of speech quality to help determine how the intensity should be adjusted for different frequency regions.

Hearing Aid Applications

So far, I have primarily used examples of tones such as those produced by a piano string and a tuning fork. In the real world, you may go days or weeks without hearing a tone; rather, you hear sounds that are combinations of many tones. The spectrum of sound is important to consider when we think about the design of hearing aids. They must react quickly to high intensity fluctuations in speech signals (not making loud sounds uncomfortable), but then return to normal amplification so that your friend's voice is loud enough for you to hear and understand. The circuit of the hearing aid must be sensitive to the entire spectrum of speech, only amplifying or compressing the portions of speech that require attention.

Another consideration is the spectrum of speech compared to the spectrum of background noise. If you've ever been involved with gardening, you'll appreciate my marigold analogy. When contained in a flower patch or in a large pot by your front door, marigolds are an attractive flower. But, when they spread with wild abandon throughout your vegetable garden, they become a weed. Such is it with speech. Most people with hearing impairment who complain of difficulty in background noise are actually complaining of difficulty in "background speech." In a crowded restaurant, for example, the majority of the noise is other people talking. Imagine how this can limit the effectiveness of even the most sophisticated digital hearing aids. A hearing aid that reduces noise will also reduce part of the speech signal. The task of the design engineer is to build a hearing aid that amplifies the speech that you want to hear but doesn't amplify the speech that you don't want to hear. The device that can do that most effectively is our brain. So, one hearing aid fitting strategy is to make all sounds audible, clear, and undistorted, and then let your brain do what it does better than an electronic circuit, process speech.

Transmission of Sound through the Ear

The transmission of sound through the pathways of the ear is a remarkable process, and the complexity of the human body is beautifully represented in the mechanics of this journey. Figure 3-2 shows the various parts of the ear.

The Outer Ear

The outer ear, referred to as the pinna is no doubt the part of the ear with which you are the most familiar, as you see it and touch it every day. We know that the outer ear has some very useful purposes, such as supporting eyeglasses and earrings, but there also are some acoustic advantages of the outer ear. One advantage is that the shape

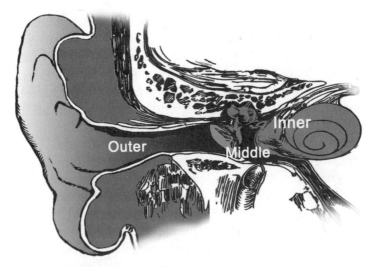

Figure 3-2: The three parts of the ear.

of the ear helps gather sound (primarily high frequencies) and channel these sounds to the ear canal. The effect is relatively small (unless your ears are much bigger than average). Not too long ago, a patient with a fairly significant hearing loss tried to convince me that when he put his hands behind his ears he could hear normally. He then asked if I didn't have a device that had big flaps on a headband that he could buy. (I guess his arms were getting tired.) When I told him I didn't, but I did have hearing aids that fit completely in the ear canal, and didn't require a headband, he left in disappointment.

The outer ear also assists in the localization of sounds, primarily differentiating sounds originating from the front and back. Some animals, of course, can maneuver their outer ears to assist them in identifying and locating different sounds. Evolution has determined that this ability is unnecessary for humans (except for everyone's Uncle Charlie, who likes to wiggle his ears to impress the children during Thanksgiving dinner). In general, although the outer ear does provide a slight loudness boost, it doesn't contribute as much to hearing as you might think. In fact, if your outer ear were completely absent, you could still have normal hearing.

Common Problem

- Infection: The outer ear can become infected, which will cause swelling and pain. This will have little or no effect on your hearing, but these infections can quickly spread to other regions, so expeditious treatment is recommended.

The Ear Canal

Once sound leaves the outer ear it enters the ear canal. The average ear canal is about 25 mm (1 inch) long. Usually, the ear canal isn't very straight. This is a good thing, as it helps prevent foreign objects from finding a direct path to the eardrum. It also helps to keep the temperature and humidity at the eardrum relatively independent from environmental conditions. Rumor has it that over thousands of years of evolution, individuals from warmer climates have developed straighter ear canals than people from cold climates—something to check out on your next trip to Antarctica!

So, how does the ear canal contribute to our hearing ability? It provides acoustic advantages, in that it is a tube, it has a resonant frequency. If you've ever blown into a bottle or other container to make it whistle, you understand the resonant frequencies of tubes. The ear canal resonance provides a boost of 10-15 dB in the 2000-3000 Hz region. This is important because as shown in Figure 3-1, these are the speech frequencies that are the softest. This boost from the ear canal is our natural "hearing aid" for understanding soft speech.

A discussion of the ear canal would not be complete without mention of "cerumen," more commonly known as earwax. It's one of those things that we usually don't talk a lot about, although it really should be considered a good friend. The purpose of earwax is to provide protection in the ear canal to dissuade invaders from finding their way to the eardrum. Invaders could be dirt, debris, or even the more unthinkable...insects. If earwax is basically good, why do people spend so much time trying to remove it? I've seen patients sitting at my desk, stick a car key or paper clip into their ear canal in search of wax. If that's what they do while I'm watching, I fear what happens in the privacy of their home! If you do happen to have a problem of too much earwax, see your physician and inquire if in your situation it's safe to flush it out with an ear lavage kit, or even under a shower head. Save your bobby pins and toothpicks for their designed purposes.

Common Problems

- Infections: The ear canal can become infected, which will cause swelling and soreness. Quite frequently, the infection is caused by someone putting something sharp in the ear canal, causing a small laceration.
- Impacted cerumen: Some people produce a great deal of earwax,

and for a variety of reasons, the wax will build up in the ear canal. On occasion, the build-up is so great that it completely occludes the canal, which will cause a mild, temporary hearing loss (it's like wearing an earplug). This wax needs to be cleaned out by a trained practitioner. Sometimes, when people first start using hearing aids, they notice a greater production of earwax—the ear canal views the hearing aid as an invader.

The Eardrum

The eardrum, more appropriately called the tympanic membrane (or TM in professional lingo), separates the ear canal from the middle ear cavity. The TM, which has a diameter of about 8-10 mm and a mass of about 14 mg, is composed of three thin layers. It is a continuously growing membrane. If you place an ink mark on one side, over a period of weeks, you'd observe it moving toward the side until it virtually rolled away on old tissue. Because most ear canals are not straight, and because it gets dark at the end of the ear canal, it's difficult to see the eardrum without using a special instrument called an otoscope. Trained practitioners can detect pathology of the eardrum (or the middle ear cavity) by observing its condition.

Like the ear canal, the eardrum serves a protective function, preventing foreign materials and climate conditions from reaching the sensitive membranes of the inner ear. Many people after swimming complain that they have "water in the ears," and some go through unusual contortions to try to remove it. Assuming that the person has an intact eardrum, this sensation is the result of water which has collected near the eardrum, and a back-pressure is preventing it from flowing out of the canal. If there were a hole in the eardrum, this water could enter the middle ear cavity, and potentially cause an infection.

The eardrum has an important auditory function, in that it helps transfer air vibrations to fluid vibrations. If airborne sound, like the sound in the ear canal, would strike a fluid like that found in the inner ear, over 99 percent of the sound energy would be reflected away. Because the inner ear depends on fluid displacement, there needs to be a way to effectively transmit sound waves to the fluid. Three bones in the middle ear cavity (we'll talk about these bones in the next section) connect the eardrum directly to one of the two membranes of the inner ear. Therefore, if a sound causes the eardrum to vibrate 500 times/second, the membrane of the inner ear will vibrate 500 times/second, which in turn causes a corresponding waveform within the fluid of the middle ear. The pressure at the inner ear is 17 times greater than at the eardrum. This is because the area of the TM is much bigger than the area of the inner ear membrane. In this way, sound is conducted by an effective method of transference of energy. Think about pounding in a nail. The aerial ratio of the head of the nail and the hammer is much greater than the point of the nail, which makes it relatively easy to transfer the necessary energy to the point. Try pounding in a nail head first, and it becomes much harder to do.

Common Problems

- Retraction: If air pressure is not equalized in the middle ear, negative middle ear pressure can develop, which causes the eardrum to retract. In this position, it doesn't vibrate as well, and a slight decrease in hearing can be noticed.
- Perforation: Any hole in the eardrum is referred to as a perforation. Most commonly, this is caused by middle ear infections or fluid in the middle ear cavity. Perforations, of course, easily can be caused by shoving objects down the ear canal. (Yes, there are hundreds of cases of eardrum perforations caused by cotton swabs.) Depending on the size and location of the perforation, there could be little or no hearing loss, or a decrease of 25-30 dB; it may heal on its own, or require surgical treatment.

Middle Ear

The middle ear is an air-filled cavity within our skull that is lined with mucus and about 2-cc in size. As we mentioned earlier, there are three bones connected to one another to form a chain between the eardrum and the inner ear. The first bone (the largest) is attached to the eardrum and is called the malleus (hammer). The next bone is the incus (anvil) and the third and smallest bone, attached to the membrane of the inner ear, is the stapes (stirrup). Several ligaments and two muscles support these three bones in the middle ear cavity.

The bones of the middle ear transfer energy from the tympanic membrane to the membrane of the inner ear (referred to as the oval window). The muscles of the middle ear also serve an auditory function. They contract when loud sounds are present, which stiffens the chain of the three bones, and causes loud sounds to be softer.

Common Problems

- Fluid Collection: Referred to as middle ear effusion; if the pressure in the middle ear is not equalized for long periods of time, fluid from the mucus membrane lining can collect in the ear. This is very common with young children. It usually causes a low frequency hearing loss (below 1500 Hz) of 15-25 dB.
- Infection: Fluid collected in the middle ear often becomes infected. When untreated, this can cause damage to middle ear structures; hearing loss usually is 20-30 dB.
- Otosclerosis: Although not as common as many other problems, you probably have heard of someone who had surgery on the "bones" of the ear and then could hear better. Sometimes there's an ossification (bony growth) around the stapes, referred to as otosclerosis, which prevents it from vibrating properly. A surgical procedure called a stapedectomy replaces the stapes and allows for improved vibrations to the inner ear.

Eustachian Tube

I've mentioned already the importance of maintaining normal atmospheric pressure in the middle ear cavity. Whether or not this happens is the responsibility of the eustachian tube, which extends from the middle ear space to the back of the throat. The tube is normally closed, but should open naturally when you talk, chew, swallow, or yawn. Whenever it opens, pressure is equalized on both sides of the eardrum. Because this tube is oriented at a downward angle, it serves a second function of allowing drainage of any excess fluid from the middle ear. In young children, the tube, not yet fully developed, is essentially horizontal—one reason why middle ear problems are more prevalent in this population.

So, what happens when the tube doesn't open as often as it should? You've probably experienced this while driving in the mountains, or descending in an airplane. If the air pressure in the middle ear cavity isn't equalized, you'll feel the external air pressure on your eardrum, and it will become retracted. You'll probably have a slight hearing loss and your own voice will sound hollow or have an echo. Young children often have a poorly functioning eustachian tube, and the pressure on the eardrum can be quite painful. This is why you'll often hear young children crying on the decent in an airplane.

The easiest way to force open your eustachian tube is to hold your nose shut with your thumb and fingers, and then try to blow air out of your nose. This is called the Valsalva maneuver. Since air cannot go out your nose, this procedure will force open your eustachian tubes (assuming that they're healthy), and will equalize middle ear pressure. If you can't do this procedure (and some people can't), exaggerated opening of the mouth might also do the trick, but be prepared for some strange stares on the airplane.

For the most part, the eustachian tube does not affect your hearing directly, except in one instance. If your eustachian tubes are not opening regularly, you may have observed that upon yawning or chewing, you suddenly were able to hear better or louder. This may last for a minute or so, and is the result of your eustachian tube opening and then slowly closing. Some people who use hearing aids are from time to time mystified how their devices can suddenly give them a "blast of clarity," and then it's gone. This is the reason.

Common Problem

- Continually closed tube: If the eustachian tube does not open because of infection or swelling, negative middle ear pressure will develop (the mucous lining of the middle ear needs air). This will cause a retraction of the tympanic membrane and eventually fluid will be drawn out of the mucous lining into the middle ear space. This fluid can become infected.

Inner Ear

We've found our way through the middle ear cavity where now entry into the inner ear occurs at the oval window, the receiver of vibrations from the eardrum. The inner ear is a cavity within the temporal bone and is referred to as the cochlea (you will hear it pronounced both "cock'-le-a" and "coke'-le-a"—take your pick). The cochlea is shaped like a snail, and has $2^3/_4$ turns. Inside the bony structure is a membranous labyrinth surrounded by fluid that runs the distance of the cochlea. When this fluid is set into motion, there's a corresponding displacement along four rows of thousands of microscopic hair cells causing stimulation of the hair cells in a given region. For example, high frequencies (short wave lengths) cause maximum displacement near the basal turn of the cochlea near the oval window. Low frequencies (long wave lengths) cause maximum displacement near the tip of the cochlea. Each region of hair cells is responsible for neural coding of a specific frequency. Loudness is coded by the degree of displacement. The thousands of hair cells perform the function of changing a hydraulic signal (fluid displacement) to an electrical signal (auditory nerve stimulation).

In addition, the balance mechanism is part of this system. The inner ear balance system consists of three semicircular canals oriented at different angles to account for any movement of the body. Like the hearing portion of the inner ear, the balance portion also includes sensory cells that react to fluid movement. In fact, the same fluid present in the cochlea communicates with the fluid of the semicircular canals. This is one reason why it's not uncommon to have a balance problem, accompanied by a hearing loss. If the ear is not producing fluid correctly, it could affect both components of this system.

Common Problems

- Presbycusis: Like many parts of the body, there's a gradual deterioration of hair cells of the inner due to aging. As discussed in the preceding chapter by Dr. Maurer, this is referred to as *presbycusis*. There isn't much, if anything, that you can do to prevent it, so don't worry about it. (Wouldn't it be nice if research showed that a glass of wine or beer each day made it better!)

- Noise-induced: Unlike presbycusis, which under current knowledge is not preventable, the second most common cause of cochlear dysfunction is noise-induced hearing loss which is preventable. Intense over-stimulation of the microscopic hair cells causes them to tear, lose their blood supply, and eventually die. When a group of cells die in a specific region, there is no longer electrical impulses for that frequency range. This damage is usually the greatest in the higher speech frequencies. Dr. Campbell will go more in-depth on this topic in a subsequent chapter on prevention of hearing loss.

- Meniere's Disease: This is the third most common cause of cochlear hearing loss. It is associated with a dysfunction of the mechanism regulating the production and/or absorption of one of the inner ear fluids. Episodes of vertigo (dizziness) and tinnitus (ringing or buzzing in the ear) often are present, and there may also be a sensation of pressure. The hearing loss may be fluctuant and usually affects the low frequencies more than the highs. A hearing loss of 30-50 dB across all frequencies is not uncommon.

Eighth Nerve

Remember that the hair cells of the cochlea transfer hydraulic energy into electrical energy. The eighth cranial nerve receives this electoral activity from the hair cells, organizes the signal, conducts further coding, and then moves the signal quickly to the central auditory system for processing.

Problem

- <u>Tumors</u>: Tumors of the auditory nerve are rare. However, they may cause hearing loss (typically unilateral high frequency) and may be associated with other symptoms such as vertigo or tinnitus.

Central Auditory System

No matter how good your hearing or the rest of the auditory system works, signals must be interpreted by the brain. Fortunately for us, the brain does a pretty good job throughout our lives. Because there are so many brain fibers available for neural interpretation, and multiple neural pathways to the brain, it's unusual for someone to have a hearing loss only because the central auditory system is not functioning normally. What can happen, however, especially as we age, is that the brain can become poorer and poorer at separating what we *want to hear* from what we *don't want to hear*. Many young people can sit and read a book while loud music and conversations surround them. An older person might have trouble "hearing" the television if only one other person is talking.

"You only hear what you want to hear" is a common phrase echoed throughout households on Sunday afternoons everywhere. "You can always hear the number of yards needed for a first down, but when I ask you to take out the trash, suddenly you have a hearing loss!"

In the summer of 1979, I spent a two-month period in the city of San Francisco. (Didn't Mark Twain once say, "The coldest winter I ever spent was a summer in San Francisco"?) I lived in a flat on Powell Street, right on the cable car line. Every fifteen minutes, late into the night, I heard the "ding-ding" of the cable car (it tends to lose its romantic appeal around 1:00 a.m.). Fortunately, the night life in San Francisco was good, since sleep at an early hour during those first few nights was not an option. After living in the flat for six weeks, some friends came over one evening. Within a few minutes they asked, "Doesn't the dinging from the cable cars drive you crazy?" My response? "What dinging?" Did my hearing change? No. Did my brain's response to my hearing change? Absolutely! Many new hearing aid users forget that their brain also will adjust to the new sounds that they hear: the squeak of a door, the click of a switch, paper crumpling, etc. It just takes time and patience.

Common Problem

- <u>Cerebrovascular changes</u>: While this does not usually cause a significant loss of hearing *per se,* it can cause difficulty in understanding and processing speech, especially in difficult listening situations. This condition involves the blood supply to the brain, and can occur gradually over years, or in transient episodes. When it occurs suddenly, it's commonly referred to as a "stroke." Blood supply to the brain affected by any condition or disease of the body can also result in hearing loss.

Taking the First Step

So, at this point you're probably thinking, "Maybe I do have a hearing loss," and, "Maybe hearing aids would make things better...**But**..." For some people, there are a lot of "But's," so many in fact that they never take action. We all need a little encouragement at times, and it comes in different forms for different people.

I remember walking into my office a few years ago on the morning of the 5th of July and listening to a telephone message on the recorder, left the night before from a patient of mine. He stated that he wanted to come in as soon as possible and order hearing aids. I knew this patient well. I had first seen him about five years earlier, and told him he needed hearing aids. He never came back. Over the years I would run into him and his wife at social functions. He would usually avoid me, but his wife would pull me off in a corner and say, "You've got to get Jim back into your office and fit him with hearing aids."

Why did Jim call me on the 5th of July? A sudden shift in hearing? No—something even more significant for him. He had spent the 4th of July weekend with his boss and two other business associates at a golf resort. By the end of the second day, the golf course jokes were no longer about traveling salesmen, but were about Jim's misunderstanding of the punch lines. This one event prompted Jim to purchase hearing aids and he soon became a full-time user. He was an ideal candidate for the completely-in-the-canal model. This is least affected by wind noise, and helped to assure Jim that he would never miss another golf course punch line!

What do we do with the "Jim's" of the world who need a giant push rather than a simple nudge when it comes to obtaining hearing aids? One approach is to simply say, "Until they're ready, there's no use in pushing them into hearing aids." To some extent, this is true, but we must be careful in making generalizations. In 1985, I was working at Walter Reed Army Medical Center in Washington, DC. We had a clinical staff of 15 audiologists and were dispensing about 5,000 hearing aids/year; nearly all the patients were retired military individuals (mostly males) who received hearing aids free of charge. We found that over 1/3 of the patients who had hearing aid fitting appointments would state at the time of their clinic visit that they really didn't want hearing aids. In fact, if we sent them home without them, they were delighted. So why did they have appointments? Because someone (usually their wife or medical professional) told them to go to Walter Reed to obtain hearing aids. This prompted us to conduct a research project, which led to some interesting findings.

We asked each one of our patients who had never used hearing aids to tell us the primary reason why they scheduled an appointment. While there were many reasons, the majority of patients fell into one of three categories because:

1) "I'm having trouble understanding speech."
2) "A medical professional told me to make the appointment."
3) "My wife (or significant other) encouraged me to make the appointment (or, in many cases, made the appointment for me)."

Regardless of the reason, we fit everyone with hearing aids. Six months later, we mailed a questionnaire to all patients so they could rate hearing aid use and satisfaction. What group do you think *used* their hearing aids the most?—The group that obtained hearing aids because of encouragement from their wives. (Hopefully, they're also encouraging them to keep them in their ears!) What group was the most satisfied with hearing aids? Those encouraged by a medical professional. What group rated the lowest in both categories?—Those who sought hearing aids on their own (maybe their expectations were too high). So, what does this mean? This study showed that just because someone is not enthusiastic about obtaining hearing aids, they can still become a satisfied user, once given the opportunity to use hearing aids and personally experience the benefits.

Ten Myths about Hearing Loss and Hearing Aids

What are some of the things that serve as roadblocks to obtaining hearing aids? Here's a few that I hear all the time, so often in fact, that I've labeled them the ten myths of hearing loss and hearing aids.

1) I'll just have some minor surgery like my friend did, and then my hearing will be okay.

Many people know someone whose hearing improved after medical or surgical treatment, and it's true that some types of hearing loss can be successfully treated. With adults, unfortunately, this only applies to 5-10 percent of cases.

2) Everyone mumbles when they talk to me.

Yes, there are a few people who mumble (good luck trying to lip-read Barbara Walters!), but, if you think that *everyone mumbles*, it's time to realize that maybe it's you, not who's speaking.

3) My hearing loss is normal for my age.

Isn't this a strange way to look at things? But, do you know what? "Doctors" tell this to their patients everyday. It happens to be "normal" for overweight people to have high blood pressure. Does that mean that they shouldn't receive treatment for the problem? I tell my patients, "You're right, your hearing is normal for your age; most people your age have hearing loss and can be helped with hearing aids."

4) I only have hearing loss for high pitches.

High frequencies are the most important for understanding speech. This is especially true when background noise is present, because the noise (which is low frequency) masks out speech in the region of normal hearing. The result: "I can hear but I can't understand."

5) I have one ear that's down a little, but the other one's okay.

Everything is relative. Nearly all patients who believe that they have one "good" ear actually have two "bad" ears. When one ear is slightly better than the other, we learn to favor that ear for the telephone, group conversations, and so forth. It can give the illusion that "the better ear" is normal when it isn't. Most types of hearing loss affect both ears fairly equally, and about 90 percent of patients are in need of hearing aids for both ears.

6) I only need but one hearing aid.

If I'm sort of sick I take one aspirin, if I'm really sick I take two. Sorry, it doesn't work that way with hearing aids. If you only have a mild vision problem do you use a monocle? If you have a hearing loss in both ears, hearing aids should be worn in both ears—that's the way the human body was designed. Haven't you heard the saying, "Don't mess with Mother Nature"? Using two rather than one hearing aid has many advantages such as: requiring less overall power from the hearing aids, hearing people on either side of you, improved speech understanding in noise, and ability to localize sound. It's very difficult to listen with just one ear.

7) I have a "nerve" loss, my doctor said it can't be helped with hearing aids.

First, as we discussed earlier in this chapter, most people have hearing loss because of damage to the *sensory mechanism* of the inner ear (cochlea), not the auditory nerve itself. Secondly, it's precisely this inner-ear-type of disorder for which hearing aids are designed, and nearly everyone using and benefiting from hearing aids has this type of problem.

8) Hearing aids will make me look "older" and "handicapped."

Looking older is clearly more affected by almost all other factors besides hearing aids. It's not the hearing aids that make one look older, it's what they imply. If hearing aids help you function like a normal hearing person, for all intents and purposes, the stigma is removed. Hearing aid manufacturers are well aware that cosmetics are an issue to many people, and that's why today we have hearing aids that fit totally in the ear canal (essentially not noticeable unless someone is staring directly into your ear). This style of hearing aid has enough power and special features to satisfy at least 50 percent of individuals with hearing impairment. But more importantly, keep in mind that "a hearing loss is more obvious than a hearing aid." Smiling and nodding your head when you don't understand what's being said makes your condition more apparent than the largest hearing aid.

9) Hearing aids will make everything sound too loud.

Hearing aids are amplifiers. At one time, the way that hearing aids were designed, it was necessary to turn up the power in order to hear soft speech (or other soft sounds). Then, normal conversation indeed would have been too loud. With today's hearing aids, however, the circuit works automatically, only providing the amount of amplification needed based on the input level. In fact, many hearing aids today don't have a volume control.

10) I simply won't do any better when I use hearing aids.

I have never fit anyone with hearing aids who did not do better with them than without them. I have fit many people, however, who didn't do as well as they had hoped or expected. This is different. Unrealistically high expectations usually lead to dissatisfaction. For the most part, few people are dissatisfied with their hearing aids, and this has been documented in research, as you'll discover in Dr. Kochkin and Gail Gudmundsen's Chapter 5. Satisfaction does vary from one listening environment to another. For example, a study conducted in 1995 showed that when people were fitted with completely-in-the-canal hearing aids with automatic signal processing, only 1-3 percent were dissatisfied when listening to television or in small groups, and 10 percent were dissatisfied when listening in restaurants. The lowest satisfaction was listening in large groups, where 15 percent of people said they were dissatisfied with their hearing aids in this environment. Two things to keep in mind. First, most people do not spend a large part of their lives in large groups, and secondly, people with normal hearing complain *they* are dissatisfied that they can't understand better in large groups.

Did any of these myths sound familiar? If you're ready to put them behind you, then it's time to make a visit to your friendly hearing health care professional.

Closing Thoughts

Living with any imperfection of the body is not an easy thing. And of all the senses which link us in the most expressive way to other people, in a way that allows us to bring out a part of our true thoughts and feelings, hearing is it. Because its diminution occurs so slowly for most of us, by the time we realize it's happened, it's usually too late. Take careful observation of your hearing. Preserve it. Protect it. Regain that communication channel you might have lost. It's a link as nourishing as food.

CHAPTER FOUR

How to Obtain Professional Help

Robert E. Sandlin, Ph.D.

Dr. Sandlin received his Ph.D. in Clinical Audiology from Wayne State University in 1961. He serves as an Adjunct Professor of Audiology at San Diego State University. He serves as Director of the California Tinnitus Assessment in San Diego which is devoted to developing effective strategies for the nonmedical management of those with subjective tinnitus. Dr. Sandlin has published over 80 articles and edited four major texts on hearing aid sciences and amplification, and contributed a number of chapters to other texts. A source of continual, personal enjoyment for him and his wife, Joann, is the love of five children.

The task of finding the most qualified individual to manage whatever hearing problems you have is not as difficult as it might first seem. Your biggest challenge will probably be narrowing your search down from a multitude of choices to a few options. In doing so, you'll minimize your potential frustrations and sharpen your focus on what's required.

As aptly described in previous chapters, many individuals find it difficult to admit to the existence of hearing impairment great enough to interfere with the understanding of speech. Hearing loss can diminish both the enjoyment of social contact as well as the ability to carry out simple tasks which merely require understanding of a command or verbal direction. Equally as important is the realization that hearing loss can create feelings of doubt about your ability to function adequately in a society where verbal communication is such an essential asset. Hearing impairment can alter family relationships and needlessly disrupt their harmony.

The purpose of this chapter is to suggest positive steps you may take in finding effective resolution to your hearing problem. One realizes this it's difficult at times to take definitive action regarding a personal problem. It's a frequent human characteristic to postpone doing something until the need is so evident that action *must* be taken. Please consider the following as a reasonable path to follow in seeking a bridge into hearing health care management.

Obviously, one of the first steps to be taken is admitting to yourself that a problem exists. Until you're ready to investigate possible solutions to your hearing problem, little of substance can be accomplished. Let's assume that you're now willing to investigate causes underlying your loss of hearing, as well as procedures which can be followed to restore your communication skills to the best which may be attained.

This chapter will go into length on several key issues which should provide meaningful guidance to you and your family. In the process, I hope it will reduce your fears, apprehensions and frustrations so often associated with any search for effective ways to manage a health problem. By the end of this chapter, you should be knowledgeable about how to move through the maze of hearing health care professionals. You should know who's who in our profession. You should be able to establish who is the best person to meet your particular needs. You will know how to determine the qualifications of the provider who might best serve you.

History of Hearing Aid Dispensing

In the early days of hearing aid dispensing, there was no sophisticated diagnostic or hearing aid measuring equipment to validate the degree of improvement provided by hearing aids or to qualify their acoustic performance. As a result of poor and sometime even improper selection and fitting procedures, some negative attitudes were developed by those who had less than positive experiences with their hearing aids. Much of this dissatisfaction was also due to rather crudely developed amplification equipment, and the lack of knowledge available to dispensers at that time. However, it's important for you to know that significant and positive changes have come about within the hearing aid dispensing field. As the manufacturing of hearing instruments has become more technologically advanced, so has the ability to measure their electroacoustic characteristics. Furthermore, many manufacturers have initiated training programs which have improved the quality of consumer care.

By the 1970's, most individuals who dispensed hearing instruments were licensed by the state in which they practiced. In order to receive a hearing aid dispensing license, a comprehensive test of basic competency had to be passed. Today, these tests have become more sophisticated and include such areas as anatomy, physiology and neurology of the auditory system; factors contributing to hearing impairment; psychology of the hearing impaired person; electroacoustic properties of hearing aids; electroacoustic measurement of hearing aid devices; administering and understanding hearing tests;

understanding and employing audiometric test results for the purpose of fitting hearing aids; learning effective counseling strategies; and becoming familiar with state laws governing the professional activities of hearing instrument providers. It can be stated with considerable assurance that anyone dispensing hearing aids today is far more qualified to select and fit these devices than they were at any time in the past. This qualification has been largely based on state licensure and mandatory continuing education requirements.

Presently, there are two individual and distinct disciplines now dispensing hearing aids: the hearing instrument specialist (HIS), and the clinical audiologist. Both can be equally qualified for the purpose of dispensing hearing aids, although their training originates from two entirely separate paths.

Hearing Instrument Specialists

There are thousands of qualified hearing instrument specialists throughout the United States. State requirements and licensing assures that they are knowledgeable and capable of performing necessary measurements to select the most appropriate hearing instruments. Many are members of the International Hearing Society (IHS). In order to qualify for membership in this group, continuing education is mandatory. The IHS also provides additional training to achieve Board Certification (BC) status. In order for members to be board certified, a written examination must be taken and passed. This examination is more demanding of specific knowledge than is the examination of individual states.

Clinical Audiologists

The advanced training and educational requirements (minimum of a Master's Degree, typically six years) of clinical audiologists primarily lends itself to the diagnostic procedures required to differentiate various pathologies of the auditory system. This may include anything from wax in the ear to a tumor resting on the eighth nerve. In addition to courses in hearing aid dispensing procedures, advanced rehabilitation courses are offered. The governing body for clinical audiologists is the American Speech, Language and Hearing Association (ASHA) which issues certification for audiology practice after extensive clinical training and passing a national exam which leads to the Certificate of Clinical Competence (CCC). Inclusion of hearing aid dispensing as an integral part of an audiology practice began in the early 1980s and has continued to grow.

The Preferred Dispensing Professional

Whether your provider is a clinical audiologist or a hearing instrument specialist, he or she must pass the same mandatory state examination and complete the required number of continuing education hours each year to maintain licensure. Members of both groups must abide by the same standards of ethical practice and are subject to the same state laws governing the dispensing of hearing aids. Each group has access to most of the same hearing instrument manufacturers and to all literature and clinical information pertaining to hearing aids and their electroacoustic performance. There are no restrictions placed on which manufacturer can provide the hearing aid device to those who dispense. All practitioners have access to pertinent scientific and trade journals and may very well modify their practice of selection and fitting of hearing aids based on current information and knowledge gleaned from specific articles.

In the selection of a qualified provider, you want someone who has demonstrated proficiency and competence. You must realize that you'll be using hearing aid amplification for many years to come, and therefore, will want to establish a long-term relationship with whomever you choose. This is something to which you should give considerable thought.

So, at this point in your reading, you may very well ask the question; "To whom do I go to receive the best possible care for my particular hearing impairment?" This is an honest question and one that deserves a straightforward and extended answer. Listed below are some of the recommended criteria to be used in selecting the best person in whom you can place confidence and trust.

Years Of Service

If somebody has been providing hearing services for many years, it generally is an indicator that many people with hearing loss have been served. This suggests that this person has been in business awhile and is likely to remain in business for the foreeable future. As with any skill-related work, the longer you do it, the more proficient you become. In the selection process, you may want to determine the years of service a particular practitioner has in providing amplification devices to those with hearing loss.

Level Of Knowledge

It's in your best interest to determine the level of skill one has in the selection and fitting process. As with any practitioner in any field, some individuals will excel at their work; others may fall short. In the past decade, there have been significant changes in this industry every few years. You should not feel uncomfortable, and the provider should not feel challenged, if you inquire about his or her level of knowledge as it pertains to current hearing aid selection and use. As a matter of fact, many hearing instrument providers may display a variety of certificates indicating they've taken specific courses of study to become more competent in selected dispensing areas. You should take advantage of this by carefully noting the dates on these displayed certificates. If you observe no continuing education courses within the past year, you might want to inquire about such recent studies.

Empathy

Knowledge of hearing aid dispensing is fundamental to doing business. But the temperament and likability of the one with whom you are doing business cannot be regulated by a state agency. Like a physician with good bedside manners, you want a professional who conducts himself or herself in a way that allows you to feel protected. You want this person to be sensitive and compassionate. You want to be able to feel comfortable revealing your very private feelings regarding hearing aid use. You don't want to feel like you're intruding, but rather, like this professional appreciates the opportunity to serve you. It's in your best interest to gather a good sense about the person with whom you are expected to work closely.

Talk to Successful Hearing Aid Wearers

It was stated earlier in this chapter that all hearing losses are not the same. Regardless of the degree and type of hearing loss you may have, others with permanent hearing loss can tell you of their experiences with a given practitioner and whether or not they were satisfied with the services offered and the benefits received. Ask people who have utilized hearing aids for several years. They have experienced the contributions and limitations of technological advances in hearing aid design and performance. They can be a rich resource for you.

Background Check

As would be true in any profession, if you're uncertain about the professional providing service to you, contact the Better Business Bureau in your community or directly contact the State committee responsible for hearing aid licensure. You may also check with the IHS or ASHA (listed in Chapter 14). Further, in some states, the association of hearing aid dispensers will have an Ethics Committee. By contacting this committee, you can ascertain if complaints have been registered against a given provider and how such complaints were resolved.

Avoid "Spur Of The Moment" Decisions

At times, people who have decided to proceed with a hearing aid evaluation and subsequent hearing aids, may consult the yellow pages and select the individual whose advertisement is most visually attractive or largest. Others may select the first business beginning with "A." It could be just as prudent to follow the suggestions given above prior to making a firm decision, although such advertising may certainly reveal special qualifications of the practitioner you are considering. Furthermore, if you feel pressured to make a decision that you might later regret, give serious thought to your feelings. On the other hand, do not compromise the help you actually need by abandoning the search.

Medical Practitioners

Many people prefer to begin their hearing health care journey with the family physician who they've known for years and who's judgment they trust. This family practitioner can then make a referral to a hearing aid provider or, if something about the ears is in need of particular attention, you could be referred to a medical specialist whose primary concern is the diagnosis and treatment of impaired hearing and diseases of the ear. Such a specialist is an otologist. An otolaryngologist is a specialist of the ear, nose and throat (ENT physician). While either can provide you with adequate treatment, otologists are even more specialized in their training.

If your physician or medical specialist refers you to someone for hearing aids, it should be safely assumed that the practitioner knows you will receive competent care. If you have any doubts about such a referral, you should ask your physician whatever questions are on your mind.

The Medical Waiver

If you're an experienced hearing aid user and you're being issued another set of hearing aids, federal law does not mandate that you be seen by a physician. This is because the government takes for granted that by now you're experienced enough to recognize the presence of a problem which needs medical attention. New users may not be as knowledgeable. In light of potential problems, federal law requires that anyone dispensing hearing aids be able to recognize a number of fairly obvious conditions of the ears. (See Chapter 9, Q/A #6 for further information.) If a medical condition is recognized by your provider, you can be assured that you'll be referred for treatment prior to issuance of hearing aids (experienced users as well).

If you're a first-time hearing aid user, federal law allows you to visit a hearing aid provider without first being seen by a physician, so long as you sign a *waiver of medical evaluation for hearing*. This essentially states, "You are being advised that the Food and Drug Administration has determined that your best health interests would be served if you had a medical evaluation by a licensed physician prior to purchasing hearing aids."

The waiver serves two solid purposes. First, it alerts you, the consumer, to the fact that a potentially serious medical problem could exist, and should not be overlooked, especially if you have any ear symptoms. Second, if you were recently seen in a physician's office and you know there's nothing wrong with your ears (other than hearing loss), you shouldn't have to go back through the medical route to obtain approval for a hearing aid purchase. Many consumers feel that a medical visit under these circumstances is both unnecessary, even redundant, and simply adds to the cost. By signing the waiver, you exercise the right to make your own decision.

A Hearing Evaluation

There are a number of procedures which a clinical audiologist or hearing instrument specialist can do to determine the magnitude of your hearing disorder. Please keep in mind that all tests administered are necessary in order to make the most appropriate assessment of your needs and determine the best approach to your subsequent care. In essentially all cases, there's no pain or discomfort involved during the administration of diagnostic tests.

Otoscopic Examination

Prior to the administration of possibly several tests, your hearing health care provider should perform a routine otoscopic examination. Its purpose is to visually examine the status of your ears. It takes less than a few minutes to complete and adds greatly to the proper diagnosis of your hearing impairment. To do this, an otoscope is used. It's a hand-held instrument about the size of a small flashlight which casts a sharply focused bright light down the ear canal and reveals the condition of the ear canal as well as anatomical structures of the eardrum. The otoscope magnifies these structures and allows visualization of potentially any abnormal condition contributing to your hearing impairment. For example, edema (swelling) of the outer ear may be seen. It some cases, it narrows the ear canal enough that it prevents sound from getting through at a normal loudness level. Otoscopic examination can also determine if a build-up of earwax is blocking sound from entering the ear. Naturally, the greater the skill and training of the professional performing the otoscopy, the greater the chances are that a problem will be recognized.

One of the major contributions of an otoscopic examination is that of assessing the status of the eardrum. For example, there could be a hole in the eardrum due to some traumatic incident or disease process. The size and impact of the hole would have to be evaluated. Further, otoscopic examination can detect the presence of fluid in the middle ear space. Its effect on your ability to hear varies with the amount of fluid and its viscosity (consistency).

Listening for Tones

Following otoscopic examination, a number of specialized hearing tests may be conducted. The purpose of hearing tests is to determine how much hearing loss you have, if any, and what is the probable cause. Usually, the basic hearing test consists of sitting in a sound-treated chamber, listening to a series of tones, and indicating to the professional when you've heard them. Some tones will be low frequency (pitch) and others will be high. As you know by now, if you have a hearing loss, you won't be able to hear all of the tones at normal intensity levels, nor will you know how well or poorly you've done until the test is completed.

The lowest tones which the human ear can detect are very close to the sensation of touch or feeling. At the other end of the continuum, a young healthy person can hear tones even higher than the highest violin note. We don't actually need to hear at either of these two extremes, but we do need hearing intact in the middle range where speech sounds vibrate. As discussed in earlier chapters, most people have greater difficulty hearing high frequencies. This is readily demonstrated by listening to (without looking at) someone repeat vowel sounds which are all low frequency, such as /a/, /e/, /i/, /o/ and /u/. Now have them produce the utterance of higher frequency sounds which make up consonants like /sh/, /ch/ and /s/ for example. Sixty-five percent of audible speech intelligibility comes from consonant sounds. Putting all of this in context, have someone repeat the words /sheath/, /cheap/ and /sheet/. If you can't discriminate the very subtle differences between these words, you will readily appreciate and recognize how important every sound is in adding information to what you hear. You might now also suspect a high frequency loss.

Listening for Speech

Obviously, there's a direct correlation between the magnitude of your hearing loss and your ability to understand words when presented at normal speech levels. Therefore, a couple of tests will be performed to assess your ability to understand selected words. The Speech Reception Threshold (SRT) test entails repeating bisyllabic (two syllable) words such as "hot dog," "baseball," or "downtown." On this particular test, the more familiar you are with the words, the more accurate the results (you just won't be able to predict which order the words will come). These words are presented at progressively weaker volume levels until you're forced to guess at what you think the words are. The value of this test is to determine how soft certain words can be made before you can only repeat them correctly 50 percent of the time. This point is called threshold. It's used as a working reference for the amount of power that eventually will be needed in your hearing aids, and can allow a certain degree of predictable success you may have in their use.

Another test is the Word Discrimination Score. Fifty monosyllabic (one syllable) words such as "wet," "chew," and "car," are presented for you to repeat. The lower your score, the greater your difficulty in hearing and understanding people who talk with you. Usually a score poorer than 88 percent would indicate that you have at least some difficulty in some situations. None of the words on this test will be repeated if you miss them. They reflect on how you might hear under ideal listening conditions.

Assessment of Middle Ear Structures

In a complete diagnostic evaluation of your impaired hearing, other tests may be carried out to determine how well your hearing system is performing. Typically, these tests are conducted by clinical audiologists. Sometimes it's important for your practitioner to know if the eardrum is moving appropriately when sounds strike it. If some disease or pathology affects the way in which the eardrum moves, then we want to be able to identify and measure it. Such measurement is called tympanometry. A special piece of diagnostic equipment is used to accomplish this. The procedure consists of applying alternating air pressure in the outer ear canal. As pressure goes from positive to negative, the eardrum moves either in or out. Failure of the eardrum to move normally has direct clinical implications and may add a great deal of information to the final diagnosis of your hearing problem.

The audiologist may perform a special test called the acoustic reflex. To understand the importance of this test, you should know that there's a small muscle (stay peed' ius) attached to a small bone in the middle ear called the stapes (stay' peez). The stapes is one of three small bones in the middle ear. Each of these bones is connected to the other. One of these connected bones is called the malleus, which is physically attached to the eardrum. When sounds of certain loudness strike the eardrum, the muscle attached to the stapes rapidly contracts. In that the muscle is attached to the stapes and the stapes is connected to the other middle ear bones, it causes the malleus to pull inward on the eardrum, which creates a resistance of movement. This resistance is a protective mechanism. It is protective because it prevents some very loud sounds from damaging the inner ear structures. Its contraction is called an acoustic reflex, and in the event your audiologist suspects anything to be out of the ordinary, it provides very important information about the integrity of the middle ear chamber.

If these basic hearing tests confirm a loss of hearing or abnormal function, then further testing, including x-rays, blood samples, or certain brain function tests may be conducted to gain even more specific information about your hearing problem and what may be done about it. The purpose of these various tests is to compare your results with those of normal hearing persons. By making this comparison, your practitioner can quickly determine if you have normal or below normal hearing. Since you might have already suspected a hearing problem anyway, it's quite possible that these tests will confirm your suspicions. Even though some people are apprehensive in general about taking tests, let me assure you that these diagnostic procedures can be critical to arriving at a competent diagnosis of your hearing problem and its proper management.

Medical and/or Surgical Treatment

In many cases, hearing tests along with other information your practitioner establishes may indicate the need for medical or surgical management. For the most part, this is good news, for it means that such intervention could resolve your problem and restore your hearing to a normal, or near-normal state. If such is the case, there is usually no need for hearing aids. However, let's assume you have seen the ENT physician or otologist and are told that nothing medically or surgically can be done to treat your hearing problem. What can you do to improve your ability to hear and understand? Hearing aids are the recommended choice.

Conclusion

Regardless of what you may have heard from others, today's hearing health care professionals are well-trained and capable of providing competent services. Do not be misled or unduly and easily influenced by those who have had limited success. Remember that the magnitude and type of hearing loss differ from person to person. It's essential that you determine who can best care for your personal needs. Hopefully, you are now at the stage where your search for guidance has led you to accept the value and need for a hearing evaluation and possibly amplification, and you're ready to proceed.

In the final analysis, it must be you who initiates the process of help. The first step in receiving help is looking for it. And little help can be offered if you fail to deal honestly with the problem. Be assured that you'll be rewarded in your willingness to use amplification by significantly improving your ability to understand much more of your acoustic world. Your frequent requests for repeats should be markedly fewer, and your blueprint to secure a bridge to a hearing world can at last be fulfilled.

Introduction

Section II: Hearing Aids

David Kirkwood
Editor-in-Chief, *The Hearing Journal*
New York, New York

When I was invited to write the Introduction to this section, I was naturally honored. But more than that, I was excited—excited to have an opportunity at last to temper some of the frustrations that go with my job as editor. Let me explain what I mean and why I think *my* frustrations may be relevant to you if you or someone close to you is among the more than 25 million Americans who have hearing loss.

In the seven years that I have been editing and writing articles for *The Hearing Journal* and the tens of thousands of hearing professionals who subscribe to it, I've been truly awed by the progress made in developing hearing aids that can improve the lives of the men, women and children who wear them.

Our Journal has reported on the introduction of sophisticated digitally programmable hearing aids capable of being fine-tuned to provide a specific pattern of amplification required by a particular individual. During the 1990s, we covered the invention of a style of hearing aid, the completely-in-the-canal instrument, that is so small and fits so deeply into the ear canal that it's virtually invisible. Apart from its obvious cosmetic appeal, this type of hearing aid offers significant acoustic advantages not generally found in larger styles.

Most recently we've published articles on the advent of hearing aids incorporating digital signal processing, a technology that promises to give audiologists and hearing instrument specialists greater flexibility than ever in providing consumers with solutions that are tailor-made for their particular hearing difficulties and needs.

No less important than the advances in hearing aid technology have been the strides made by our profession in developing techniques for successfully applying these advances to real people like you. In the past few years, clinicians and researchers have learned a great deal about such crucial issues as:

- measuring not only a person's hearing loss but also the *handicap* that results from the loss;
- determining the precise type and amount of amplification appropriate for an individual's hearing configuration; and
- teaching consumers how to get the maximum benefit from their hearing aids.

So, you may ask, "Where's the frustration?" Isn't it rewarding to be part of a health care field in which there are so many exciting advances? Well, yes it is. But there is one thing that really bothers me, and it unhinges a lot of people I know in this profession. Very few consumers have any idea how much help for hearing loss is available to them <u>right now</u>. We've all heard about such medical breakthroughs as heart transplants, reattachment of severed limbs, and "test tube" fertilization—procedures that most of us will never have cause to undergo. But when it comes to hearing aids, a medical device that one in ten of us could benefit from <u>today</u>, most people know very little, and what they do know is often hopelessly out of date. All too many of us still base our impression of hearing aids on what we observed 25 years ago when Grandma or Uncle Fred wore one. Chances are their hearing aids didn't work all that well.

The fact is, hearing aids and hearing care have come a very long way since then. But most consumers, even those whose hearing has deteriorated, are simply unaware of the progress that has been achieved. In my opinion, this lack of consumer awareness is the number one reason why only about one person in five who could benefit from hearing aids currently uses them. And it also helps explain why so many people *needlessly* put up with the ill effects of untreated hearing loss that are discussed earlier in this book.

There is one sure cure to the deep frustration that we in the hearing health care profession feel when we think about the millions of people who have denied themselves the benefits of hearing aids. This is to educate consumers about the importance of hearing and the effectiveness of today's hearing aids in helping people overcome hearing loss.

This book, and especially this section on hearing aids, will help provide that education. The fact that you have picked up this book and are reading this page makes me optimistic. Obviously you are interested enough and open-minded enough about hearing aids to want to learn more. In this case, you've come to the right place. The contributing authors who follow, bring a wealth of experience and expertise to the subject of hearing aids. Each of the chapters contains advice and information that will be of great value if you're a prospective hearing aid candidate.

While there's much in the chapter by Dr. Kochkin and Gail Gudmundsen that you'll find interesting, let me point out one particular section entitled, "Ensuring Hearing Aid Satisfaction." In just a few paragraphs, the authors present clear, easy-to-follow advice that can make you or someone you care about a successful hearing aid wearer.

Not everyone with a hearing loss is psychologically ready for hearing aids. But how should you and your hearing care provider decide when the time for help has arrived? Dr. Weinstein discusses two important tools designed to measure the impact of hearing loss on a particular person's life. As this chapter points out, recognizing the toll that hearing loss takes is a crucial first step toward addressing the problem with hearing aids.

The more you know about hearing aids, the better are your chances of getting, and using them successfully. For this reason I strongly recommend Dr. Sweetow's chapter. Filled with sound advice, you'll discover what you can realistically expect from new hearing aids. And since any electronic device is subject to failure eventually, Drs. Smedley and Schow provide you with tips to make hearing aid ownership as trouble-free as possible.

Rounding out this section is a lively review by Richard Carmen of the latest expertise on a range of issues. One important topic that he raises with Dr. Caccavo, also a leading audiologist, is how consumers should react to the negative experiences of others with hearing aids. She wisely points out that every hearing loss is unique. That's why if you seek help, the hearing professional you go to will design a program specifically for you. In the final analysis, she notes, it is your experience that really counts. And if you approach hearing aids with a positive attitude and a willingness to follow through with the program designed for you, the chances are excellent that you'll become one of the many successful and satisfied consumers.

CHAPTER FIVE

Why Some Consumers Reject Hearing Aids But How You Could Learn to Love Them

Sergei Kochkin, Ph.D.

Gail Gudmundsen, M.A.

Dr. Sergei Kochkin is a Director of Market Development & Market Research at Knowles Electronics and the 1997 Director of the Better Hearing Institute. He has published more than 30 papers on the hearing aid market and conducted more than two dozen studies on customer satisfaction with hearing aids. He holds a Doctorate in Psychology, an MBA in marketing, and a Masters of Science in counseling and guidance. Dr. Kochkin also maintains an interest in archeology and comparative religion, and when there's time—meditation.

Gail Gudmundsen is a clinical audiologist who has been in private practice since 1980. She received her Master's Degree in Audiology from the University of Iowa in 1973. Her experience includes clinical practice, teaching, research, and organizational leadership. She has served on the Board of Directors of six state and national audiology organizations. She served on the editorial review board of Hearing Instruments, is on the adjunct faculty of Rush University, and has authored more than 25 papers and publications.

Three major research studies in the United States indicate that there are between 25 and 28 million people with hearing loss, about one in every ten Americans. In addition, two major studies indicate that slightly more than one million of this figure are school-age children. The early identification and treatment of hearing loss in children is particularly critical since hearing is synonymous with normal development of speech.

From conversations with experts in other countries, it's generally recognized that close to 10 percent of the world's population have problems with their hearing. We happen to believe this figure may be higher because most studies don't include hearing impaired populations in institutional settings such as nursing or retirement homes, the military, and prisons. Among the elderly, hearing loss is the third most serious health issue, behind arthritis and hypertension.

*All references to "research" in this chapter refer to studies conducted and compiled by Dr. Kochkin.

The vast majority (close to 90-95 percent of people with hearing loss) can be helped by hearing aids. There have been major breakthroughs in hearing aid technology in the past 10 years, and we can now match technology with a candidate's lifestyle and communication needs. Yet, many hearing aids still end up in a drawer. The good news is that most of the problems with hearing aids have been solved, and wearers can now expect improved communication with hearing aids as the rule, not the exception.

Why do some individuals have difficulty adjusting to hearing aids while others are doing so well that people around them don't even notice they're wearing them? What's different about successful hearing aid wearers? Is there a profile of a successful hearing aid user? And why do only one in five individuals with hearing loss use hearing aids despite their proven value? Some interesting facts are now coming to light which may answer these questions.

Why Most People Reject Hearing Aids

More than 20 million people in the United States have never tried hearing aids as a solution to their hearing loss. In one research investigation, close to 3,000 individuals with self-reported hearing loss were polled regarding their reluctance to try hearing aids. Here are some of the reasons why consumers have declined to pursue them.

1) Price

Investing in hearing aids may be a difficult decision if you are not knowledgeable about the potential value they can bring to your quality of life. Recent research by the National Council on Aging demonstrated that hearing aids have a dramatic impact on nearly every dimension of the human experience.

Furthermore, the body of scientific research indicates that advanced programmable technology tends to result in greater wearer satisfaction. About 40 percent of potential hearing aid wearers have indicated they cannot afford today's modern hearing aids. For people on limited incomes, quality lower cost hearing aids as well as payment plans are available through most hearing health providers.

2) Education and Awareness

Many people aren't aware they have a hearing loss and therefore are in need of information that would help them recognize it. Most people lose hearing gradually. In most cases, it's slowly progressive. During this time, the person with hearing loss and family members learn to adapt to it, often not even realizing that they're doing this. Thus, one of the first things individuals with suspected hearing loss should do is determine if they have some of the signs of hearing loss.

3) Stigma and Cosmetics

A third reason people reject hearing aids is that close to nine million people are concerned with the stigma of hearing loss or are in a state of denial, and thus try to hide it from others. It's unfortunate, but many people, because they have less than perfect hearing, believe they are inferior, unintelligent, or simply less lovable. They believe other people will think they're getting older or will be viewed as less competent, less attractive, and so on. They have shame regarding their hearing loss. This is partly due to the fact that we live in a youth-oriented, air-brushed society where physical perfection is stressed as an important human attribute.

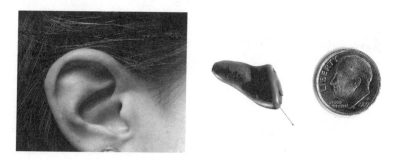

Figure 5-1: The CIC (photo right), about the size of a dime, is essentially invisible (photo left) when in the ear canal.

As you previously read in this book, cosmetics no longer need to be a barrier to obtaining amplification. Within the last few years, technological advances have permitted the hearing aid industry to develop hearing instruments like the completely-in-the-canal (CIC) devices which are essentially not very visible (See Figure 5-1). In fact, research shows that 90 percent of consumers perceive these CICs to be completely invisible. Based on your hearing needs and the physical characteristics of your ears, you might be a candidate for these "invisible devices." If you're not, rest assured that in-the-canal (ITC) devices, although larger, are available to fit many hearing losses and are not terribly noticeable. Understand though, that once you begin hearing through amplification, cosmetics will be of lesser concern to you. Research shows that people who have come to enjoy their hearing aids rate even the largest hearing aids as cosmetically appealing as compared to some of the smaller, in-the-ear models. Some hearing instruments even come in bright colors!

4) Misinformation

Many people have received misinformation about their hearing loss and the extent to which it can be helped. For instance, many physicians have recommended to their patients that they're not candidates for hearing aids if they have hearing loss in one ear and good hearing in the other; if they have "nerve deafness" (an obsolete term for sensorineural hearing loss); or if the hearing loss still allows them to conduct a conversation in quiet. Much of this misinformation has been given unintentionally by well-meaning family physicians who do not specialize in hearing problems. In fact, most physicians receive very little training in medical school in the areas of hearing loss and hearing aids.

5) Dismissing the Importance of Hearing

Another reason for rejection of hearing aids is that people have forgotten how important hearing is to their quality of life. We live in such a visually-oriented society that often, hearing plays a secondary role. As you know from your own experience, or from reading this book, people who cannot hear well, often have lives filled with anxiety, insecurity, isolation and depression. People gradually withdraw from family and friends because without auditory contact, they lose the feeling of being connected. They grow numb to the world around them. But in the world, communication is critical. We interact with one another through communication.

We're aware of a CEO who lost more than a million dollars in business because he misunderstood a client's needs. We're aware of a grandfather who was thought to be senile instead of hearing impaired. He was able to compensate for his hearing loss with hearing aids and began to effectively interact with his family again. Most hearing health care professionals know of horror stories of children being misdiagnosed as slow, retarded, hyperactive, or having poor attention spans when in fact it was impaired hearing.

6) Hearing Aids Don't Work

More than 11 million people mistakenly believe that hearing aids are not effective for what they are designed to do. Many people judge hearing aids based on what they've seen their grandparents wear—a large, clunky box about the size of a pack of cigarettes with wires coming out of it. Recent research with consumers utilizing a variety of models of hearing aids indicates that 78 percent report *satisfaction* (defined as satisfied or very satisfied) with the ability of the hearing aid to improve their hearing, while 73 percent report that hearing aids have *significantly improved the quality of their life.* If this research had been conducted 20 years ago, this remarkably high satisfaction factor probably wouldn't even be 35 percent. A significant number of people report satisfaction with their hearing aids in quiet situations (93 percent) as well as very difficult situations such as restaurants, church or large groups. Research shows that not everyone benefits equally in all listening situations, nor do all types of hearing aid circuitry perform better in difficult listening situations. As an example, the average hearing aid achieved a 29 percent satisfaction rating in noisy situations; yet some technologies, notably programmable hearing aids with multiple microphones, achieve satisfaction ratings as high as 51 percent. Similarly, only about 34 percent of consumers are satisfied with hearing aids on the telephone, yet, some instruments, such as completely-in-the-canal (CIC) hearing aids are able to *double client satisfaction* because they're located just inside the entrance of the ear canal and produce less feedback. Much of this satisfaction may also be due to diminished wind noises outdoors, a sense of more natural amplification, and the need for somewhat less power resulting in increased tolerance while in the presence of background noise.

We believe that advances in technology in just the last few years and in the near future will result in many more consumers being able to enjoy an enhanced lifestyle in increasingly difficult listening situations.

7) Trust in a Hearing Aid Dispensing Professional

The last reason why people hold off purchasing hearing aids is that nearly seven million people don't trust providers who dispense. As Dr. Sandlin describes in Chapter 4, training, education and experience among dispensers of hearing aids has greatly increased over the years for both audiologists and hearing instrument specialists. This is reflected by recent research which shows that close to *90 percent of consumers are satisfied with their hearing aid dispensing professional.* While education, knowledge and experience of dispensers varies, if you study Dr. Sandlin's chapter, you'll discover that there are some basic things you can do to assure a successful hearing aid experience. What you need to understand is that the hearing aid industry is interested in helping people hear. There could be no industry otherwise. This means striving to satisfy your highest expectations because ultimately your decision to proceed with amplification is based on the extent to which your needs will be met. Nevertheless, you must realize that to date, electronic devices for hearing cannot replace the quality of sound provided by a normal functioning ear.

Trends

We feel it would be useful to summarize the two major trends in the evolution of hearing aids over the years: *signal processing* and *size*. To an extent, this will explain why hearing aids have received such a negative image and also why this image is dramatically improving. Perhaps the image was deserved twenty-five years ago, but now there's no reason for it.

Signal Processing

In the 1960s, the best available hearing aids were limited to help in quiet only; in noise they made things worse. Therefore, it was common to have to remove them when around noise which of course resulted in not hearing well. Hearing aids of 20-30 years ago sounded like cheap transistor radios—not a very satisfying listening experience. By the 1980s, certain circuits which had become available made hearing in noise easier.

In 1997, advanced circuitry has been able to offer consumers improved quality of hearing in quiet, as well as some increased hearing ability in noise, such as in difficult listening situations like big groups, church, movies, cars, outdoors, and restaurants. Some hearing aids sample sound 50 times per second (some even faster) and selectively make loud sounds soft, and soft sounds loud. Modern-day hearing aids are effective in sending clear sound to the brain, making interpretation easier. In the past, hearing aids distorted sound. Some still do, but the best hearing aids we have now do not distort even in high noise levels.

In a Northwestern University study (Killion, 1979), it was shown that some hearing aids can produce fidelity as fine as, if not better than, expensive stereo systems. Microphones used in some hearing aids are utilized by recording and broadcast studios.

There's an incredible array of technological and cosmetic choices available to you. For instance: some hearing aids are programmable, enabling the audiologist or hearing instrument specialist to electronically adjust hearing aids to your hearing loss. If your hearing loss increases, the hearing aids can be re-programmed in your provider's office. Programmability allows you, by the push of a button, often but not always on a remote control, to gain some hearing advantages in noisier situations.

Some hearing aids have volume controls and some don't. If you have an active lifestyle or are interested in hearing aids which may not need adjustment, perhaps hearing aids which automatically adjust are most suitable for you. Other people cannot live without the flexibility of adjusting the volume on their hearing aids, so they should seek amplification which gives them this capability.

Research shows that consumers report greater satisfaction with the sound quality of today's hearing aids. They report an ability to use their hearing aids in more and more situations—even in noisy situations. This research also shows that people with hearing loss in both ears tend to be more satisfied if they use two hearing aids. The benefits of binaural hearing are most noticeable in situations where you need to be able to tell the direction of sound. Research shows that in binaural use, there's an average of a 15 percent shift in increased satisfaction when consumers are asked about their "ability to tell the direction of sounds." This is a substantial improvement! Consequently, users who wear two hearing aids tend to communicate better in their place of worship, in small group gatherings, large gatherings and even outdoors. Naturally, a person's ability to enjoy hearing aids will differ based on the specific hearing loss and the type of technology used in the hearing aids.

Size

The second major advance has been in size. Various non-electrical trumpets and horns were introduced in the 1800s. These were megaphones in reverse. Although they didn't use batteries, they offered effective but limited amplification. In fact, these are still available as a very inexpensive hearing aid, primarily in Europe. Their amplifying value would be similar to a very mild-powered hearing aid. Speaking tubes are another variation of non-electrical devices similar to the trumpet. They were used for courting, whereby individuals from a distance of three feet away could talk into the ear of a loved one without family members hearing what they had to say.

After the invention of the telephone by Alexander Graham Bell, the principle of the electrical transmission of sound was applied to hearing aids. Hearing aids were large and required carrying a battery pack strapped to your body. In the 1940s, vacuum tubes brought down the size of hearing aids to the size of a transistor radio. These are not small by today's standards, but small compared to the old electric hearing aids. It was not until the invention of transistors in the 1960s that hearing aids on the head or in the ear became available.

By reducing the size of hearing aids, people can wear them with greater comfort and we're finding very small CIC hearing aids have their distinct advantages as previously described. Some people are concerned with cosmetics and prefer the least noticeable hearing aids, in the way that you might choose contact lenses over framed eyeglasses. The problem is that the smallest hearing aid may not be the most suitable for you for a variety of reasons. Your specific hearing loss may require more power than available in CICs, or you might not have the manual dexterity to manipulate them, or your ear canals may not allow them to be retained in the ears.

What is Satisfaction?

Simply stated, satisfaction is having your expectations met—fulfillment of a promise. If this is true, then it's useful to determine what you're looking for, and most importantly, how you'll know when you've found it.

What distinguishes a satisfied hearing aid user from a dissatisfied one? Satisfied individuals believe their expectations have been met. The only way you will assure your satisfaction is to return to your provider and explain why you are not pleased. The professional is there to help you and cannot mind-read your problems in your absence. This requires steadfast willingness on your part.

Stages of Readiness

As Richard Carmen discusses in Chapter 1, change is inevitable. It's one of those constants we can count on to make life interesting (or stressful, depending on how you view it). Advanced hearing aid technology can now compensate for most hearing losses, but there are still millions of hearing aid candidates who are not ready to accept this fact. Is there a missing link? We think so. There are actual steps most people go through whenever they make changes. Examining these steps may help you understand what it takes to become a successful hearing aid user.

All of us have a different pace for readiness. Recognizing the particular stage you (or a family member) are in can help you prepare for a change which will improve your life. Acknowledging your hearing loss, and the eventual acceptance of hearing aids makes way for a healthy, productive change. Recognizing the stages of these transitions is helpful for both prospective hearing aid wearers and hearing care professionals.

Psychologist Jay Singer, Ph.D. and his colleagues* at the University of Rhode Island applied the concepts of a particular theory of behavior change to four stages of readiness that hearing aid candidates go through in the process of obtaining amplification.

1) In the first stage, the individual has <u>not accepted that there is a problem</u> and has no interest in changing. If either a family member or a professional insists on hearing aids at this point, behavior is unlikely to change.

2) In the next stage, there's <u>recognition of the hearing loss</u> and consideration of ways to change. Information is often requested about technology, circuitry options and costs. This is an important time for you to gain knowledge from the hearing care professional, discuss policies, weed out false hopes and discern realistic expectations for hearing aid use.

3) In stage three, there may still be ambivalence, but the prospective user is <u>getting ready to commit</u> to the process. There's a willingness to discuss your feelings about the problem and explore some hearing options that might be available to you.

4) Then, there's an action stage, at which time hearing aids may be purchased, but <u>actual change in behavior</u> occurs during follow-up visits, and during the adjustment and acclimatization periods that may be ongoing for several months.

Psychological Profile of a Successful Hearing Aid User

Is there a profile of a successful hearing aid user? Some interesting facts are now coming to light which may answer this question. Actually, much of this information has been with us for a long time, but we were not seeing the forest through the trees. Some of these new inferences are drawn from self-assessment scales of hearing aid

*Used by permission of the publisher, *The Hearing Review*.

benefit. While many of these tools are not new, interpretation of the data is. It's increasingly evident that there are certain personality traits common to successful hearing aid wearers, and there are certain distinguishing characteristics of hearing care providers that produce satisfied clients. Our goal is to provide you with information and insights that will result in your long-term successful and satisfied hearing aid use.

The most important personality trait that one could possess is a positive attitude, not just toward the process of obtaining hearing aids, but toward life in general. Motivation is a key to success with amplification. This means a willingness to try hearing aids, adapt to new solutions, and keep frustration at a minimum when obstacles arise. If you view your circumstances as beyond your control, there's a probability that you'll be less successful in adapting to change, including hearing aid use.

Robyn Cox, Ph.D., and her colleagues from the University of Memphis, found that personality type had an effect on hearing aid users' perceived benefit. They found that those who were outwardly oriented to the world (extroverted), who felt they were in control of their own lives, and those who had less habitual anxiety, reported greater benefit from hearing aids.

Dean Garstecki, Ph.D., from Northwestern University, recently surveyed two groups of hearing aid candidates. All received a recommendation to obtain hearing aids. Almost one-half of the group followed the recommendation and purchased hearing aids while the other half did not. They all had similar hearing losses and were in the same age range. Both groups judged themselves to be in good health.

In the area of personal adjustment, the group that wore hearing aids had a higher acceptance of their hearing loss and were less inclined to ask others to accommodate their hearing problem. They had more effective communication at home and at work, and judged the cost and visibility of their hearing aids as less important than those who did not obtain them. In addition, those who purchased hearing aids were significantly less concerned about their physician's opinion of the extent to which hearing aids could benefit them. Support and encouragement of friends and family made the biggest difference in their satisfaction.

Experienced practitioners are able to determine if your hesitation to commit to hearing aids indicates that you have not yet acknowledged the hearing loss, or if your concerns may be based on loss of self-esteem, cost, visibility of hearing aids (stigma), or further progression of hearing loss. A high level of anxiety can be reduced once the source of these concerns is established. The rehabilitative course for an outgoing individual may be quite different than for someone who may be somewhat more withdrawn, quiet and introverted. Therefore, understanding stages of change and personality of the individual leads to more effective counseling and education, and ultimately, increased consumer satisfaction.

Finally, hearing aid studies have shown that people who have a positive outlook on life do better with hearing aids. They have a positive self-image and believe they're in control of their fate. Our recommendation is take charge!

Ensuring Hearing Aid Satisfaction

There are a number of things you can do to increase the likelihood of your satisfaction with hearing aids. First, recognize that your hearing loss is making communication difficult. Accept that there's help available. It's all right to be ambivalent about the process, but be willing to seek a solution. Ask for the advice of family and friends you trust, but be careful not to dwell on negative experiences that others may have had. We frequently tell patients that we want to make them successful so that hearing aids will stop getting such a bad rap.

Identify which communication situations are most difficult for you. If you can describe difficult listening conditions, your hearing care provider can address the problems and develop strategies to help you manage them. If you need more information, ask for it. Some people want highly technical information, some just want a brief overview of hearing aids and their function. Most providers will be happy you asked, and will give you information such as consumer guides, data sheets, brochures, videotapes and other types of instructional materials. Ask for clarification if you need it. Many complex concepts can be explained in an uncomplicated way.

Be realistic. Remember that it takes time to get used to hearing aids, especially if you're a new user. Keep in mind that background noise is almost always part of your environment and adjustment to it is required. In time, you will tune out many of these everyday sounds. It's important not to become disappointed or frustrated while your brain begins to adjust to a whole new world of sound. If you're an experienced user trying new hearing aids, understand that they might not sound like your old ones. Before you reject them, allow neural hook-ups in the auditory system to adapt to these new sounds. You just might find that you like this new sound better than the old one.

Follow the instructions you're given during the initial stages of adjustment. You may need a specific wearing schedule for hearing aids. One experienced in-the-canal hearing aid user obtained CIC instruments about two years ago. He was in his early 30s and had used hearing aids since he was a teenager. When he returned for his two-week recheck, he was asked how long he could wear the instruments in the beginning. He said that he could only use them for 15 minutes at a time. Within two weeks he was wearing them full-time and they were completely comfortable. Had he not been counseled that the deep insertion of the shell tip with CICs may take extra time to fully adjust, he might have become discouraged and given up on that particular style.

Be patient with yourself. If you have the best hearing aids for your hearing loss and your lifestyle, hang in there. Make sure you're comfortable with the advice you've been given. Ask questions. Remember, your provider is your advocate.

Satisfied hearing aid users are not shy when it comes to telling others about their success, but unfortunately, neither are the ones who are not satisfied. No two people are alike, and it's not a good idea to assume that if someone has had a bad experience, hearing aids are bad. You could very well be one of the overwhelming majority who has a good experience! There are many reasons why someone may not have been successful, so don't project these conditions and improbabilities onto yourself. Also, do not expect someone else's hearing aids to work for you. Would you wear their eyeglasses and decide whether you can be helped by glasses based on this experience?

Realistic Expectations of Your Hearing Care Provider

Hearing aid researchers agree that the interaction of the provider and the client is a critical element in successful hearing aid use. There are specific elements to this important relationship that are common to providers who achieve a high degree of satisfaction among their clients. Successful providers believe in the efficacy (benefit) of hearing aids and they keep up with rapid changes in hearing aid technology.

Expect your provider to be able to explain hearing aid options to you in simple terms. Demonstrations are often helpful which allow you to listen to a particular type of circuitry, to compare different settings in noise, or to experience the difference between monaural (one hearing aid) and binaural amplification. A good professional dispensing hearing aids never assumes that clients cannot understand complex concepts. You should be given as much information as you require in the form of discussion, videotapes, brochures, consumer guides, and technical articles. Currently, there's a popular phrase, "too much information." There's also a time to stop giving information. Not all patients want or need a bus load of materials. Information needs to be tailored to your needs.

Knowing the stages of change previously discussed is useful in helping you to accept your hearing loss and move toward obtaining hearing aids. Research has identified that *stigma* is still a very common reason why people hold back from purchasing hearing aids. It's very important that you're allowed to express your feelings about how hearing aids will look and what you think about them. Simply talking about your feelings associated with your hearing loss can be of tremendous benefit. Some people don't care what size or style of hearing aid is chosen. Others are extremely conscious about the cosmetic aspect. Sociologist Dr. Cuzzart in Chapter 9 offers valuable insights on stigma.

Experienced providers know how to motivate skeptical, timid hearing aid candidates. They know that proactive clients have a higher likelihood of becoming satisfied hearing aid users. All providers want their clients to be willing to go the distance, even if they make a few mistakes in the beginning. Sometimes the process can be difficult. A caring professional will always see you through *if you will*.

Optimizing the match between your lifestyle and communication needs is an important determination by your provider, something which can have direct impact on you. We're all more likely to trust someone who we feel is compassionate and understands us. Therefore, effective hearing care providers are good listeners. It's important that your provider takes the time to learn what problems you have in meetings, groups, theater, with co-workers, family, and in your place of worship. It's also important for you to express what you hope to improve in your hearing world as a result of amplification.

Readiness

As discussed previously with respect to stages of readiness, you must reach the point in your own willingness to proceed. If given the chance to express your feelings about hearing loss, including issues of loss and self-esteem, you're most likely to make a decision at the first visit with your hearing care professional to proceed with hearing aids and are equally likely to be successful. Well-meaning family members cannot usually coerce you to receive help until you've achieved such personal resolution.

Family members who participate in your decision to seek help need to be sensitive to your readiness, and respect it. By the same token, it's essential that you do not unduly stall the process. Some people need time to accept their hearing loss, and with proper information and reassurance from an experienced provider, success will be the net result. Proactive patients who take charge of their own lives are the most successful hearing aid users.

Common Reasons for Failure

Historically, people were unsuccessful with hearing aids because there was little perceived benefit. The bandwidth was limited and fidelity was marginal. At higher volume levels, or when there was a sudden loud noise, hearing aids badly distorted or were uncomfortable. Most fittings were monaural, which severely limited the brain's ability to sort things out. And, most importantly, in the presence of noise, it was actually easier and more comfortable to hear without amplification.

All of this has changed with current technology. The major problems have been solved, and we now have hearing aids that don't produce distortion, don't require frequent volume control adjustment, and don't cause discomfort. The remaining hurdle is improved hearing in noise, which even the most sophisticated digital hearing aids cannot change unless the signal-to-noise ratio is improved. To our knowledge, the only viable techniques for improving communication in noise are hearing aids with directional microphones, or FM systems.

There's often a high degree of skepticism surrounding hearing aids, in large part because of negative attitudes from others who have tried them and were not satisfied. The challenge for today's hearing care providers is to keep up with the new technology which includes a vast array of signal processing possibilities and multiple features.

In a research study with 5,000 users, satisfaction was significantly higher among those whose hearing aids had features such as programmability, wide dynamic range compression, multiple memories, multiple channels, and directional microphones. Kenneth Dychtwald, author of *Age Wave*, and an expert in the field of aging, has proposed that to increase satisfaction with hearing aids, the hearing aid industry should remove all of the outdated hearing aids from the field. That would be a bold and expensive move, but would go a long way toward beginning the process of improving trust in hearing care providers, and would eliminate the old technology which is still causing much of the dissatisfaction among consumers.

Myths

As Dr. Mueller nicely points out in Chapter 3, there are many common myths still prevalent about hearing loss and hearing aids. Here are a few more to put in "the hopper" and dispel as we approach the 21st Century.

Your hearing cannot be helped.

In the past, many people with hearing loss in one ear, with a high frequency hearing loss, or with nerve damage have all been told they cannot be helped, often by their family practice physician. This might have been true many years ago, but with modern advances in technology, nearly 95 percent of people with a sensorineural hearing loss can be helped by hearing aids.

Hearing loss affects only "old people" and is merely a sign of aging.

Fewer than 40 percent of people with hearing loss are older than age 64. There are close to eight million people in the U.S. between the ages of 18 and 44 with hearing loss, and more than one million are school-age.

If I had a hearing loss, my family doctor would have told me.

Not true! Only 16 percent of physicians routinely screen for hearing loss during a physical. Since most hearing impaired people hear well in a quiet environment like your doctor's office, it can be virtually impossible for your physician to recognize the extent of your problem. Without special training in, and understanding of the nature of hearing loss, it may be difficult for your doctor to even believe that you have a hearing problem at all.

The consequences of hiding hearing loss is better than wearing hearing aids.

At what price vanity? We go back to the old adage that a hearing loss is far more noticeable than hearing aids. If you miss a punch line to a joke, or respond inappropriately in conversation, people may wonder what's going on with you. The personal consequences of vanity can be life-altering. It means giving up some portion of the sounds you used to enjoy. In the end, it's really not worth giving up on your hearing.

I'll wait until technology improves.

If you've read this far in this book already, then by now, you should know the answer to this one! Technology has improved and is waiting for you! On a trial basis, what do you have to lose?

References

Cox, R.M., Alexander, G.C., Grey, G.A. Relationships between selected personality variables and self-assessed hearing aid benefit. American Academy of Audiology Annual Convention Poster Session. Salt Lake City, Utah, 1996.

Dychtwald, K. *Age Wave*. New York: CG Putnam & Sons, 1989.

Garstecki, D.C. & Erler, S. Counseling of older adult hearing instrument candidates. High Performance Hearing Solutions, Vol. 1, January, 1997.

Garstecki, D.C. Older adults: hearing handicap and hearing aid management. American Journal of Audiology, Vol 5 (3), 25-33, 1996.

Killion, M.C. Design and evaluation of high fidelity hearing aids. Doctoral thesis, Northwestern University. Ann Arbor: University Microfilms, 1979.

Singer, J., Healey, J. and Preece, J. Hearing instruments: a psychological & behavioral perspective. High Performance Hearing Solutions, Vol. 1, January, 1997.

CHAPTER SIX

From Hearing Loss to Hearing Aids: Bridging the Gap

Barbara E. Weinstein, Ph.D.

Dr. Weinstein is a Professor of Audiology and Program Director at Lehman College, City University of New York (CUNY), and is on their doctoral faculty at the Graduate School and University Center. She's the recipient of the 1996 Distinguished Clinical Achievement Award from the New York State Speech-Language-Hearing Association. She's authored over 40 manuscripts on hearing loss and hearing aids in adults, and is co-author of the Hearing Handicap Inventory for Adults and the Elderly. Dr. Weinstein is editor of several books on hearing loss in the elderly; and is currently completing a textbook on hearing loss, hearing aids and the elderly

The problems that result from a hearing impairment can be described in terms of the self-perceived disabling or handicapping effects. The extent of disability is defined by the auditory difficulties in a variety of listening situations as perceived by the person with hearing impairment. These might include difficulty understanding television, the clergy at a religious service, friends in a restaurant, and so forth. "Handicap" represents the non-auditory problems (such as isolation, loneliness, confusion) resulting from diminished auditory capacity. Disability and handicap are typically quantified using questionnaires which require respondents to answer questions about how they perceive the hearing loss to be affecting them. Responses to self-report questionnaires provide information from the client's perspective about the problems associated with hearing impairment. Responses to questions on the scales help hearing health care professionals quantify social and emotional consequences of hearing loss, suggest the impact of these changes on independence and quality of life, set the objectives or goals of the intervention program, and define the criteria against which success of a rehabilitation program will be judged. With regard to hearing aid fittings, the magnitude of change in the client's self-reported disability or handicap is currently being used to infer the benefits provided by hearing aids.

Recently, it has come to the attention of hearing care professionals, namely audiologists, that the patient's perception and acceptance of the fact that hearing loss exists, is the motivating factor behind a referral for assistance. In fact, the U.S. Public Health Service recommends that adults should routinely be questioned about signs of hearing loss to ascertain the need for some form of intervention. Questionnaires have the advantage of identifying people who perceive hearing loss to be a problem and who therefore may be particularly motivated to use hearing aids. They strongly recommend that people found to have evidence of hearing loss by screening be considered for referral to a specialist for comprehensive audiological evaluation, especially if you feel handicapped by hearing loss. The Public Health Service suggests that a reliable and valid screening questionnaire may be used to screen for social, emotional, and communication handicaps stemming from hearing loss.

Two simple, reliable and valid screening tools, namely, the 10-item screening (symbolized by "-S") versions of the Hearing Handicap Inventory for Adults (HHIA-S) or for the Elderly (HHIE-S) have gained widespread acceptance among physicians, nurses, nurse practitioners, and audiologists. The HHIA-S is primarily for individuals under 65 years of age because it was initially standardized on this population. The HHIE-S was standardized on adults over 65 years of age and is hence more appropriate for them. The purpose of the items comprising the questionnaires, which are shown in Tables 6-I and 6-II, is to identify persons with handicapping hearing impairment who require audiological testing and are likely to purchase and benefit from hearing aids and/or assistive listening devices.

Each of the questionnaires can be completed using a paper and pencil, or by computer-assisted presentation, or by having someone orally ask you the questions. As is evident from Tables 6-I and 6-II, the HHIE-S and HHIA-S, respectively, consist of two types of questions, namely social (S) and emotional (E). The five social questions attempt to isolate your self-perceived difficulties in a given situation whereas the five emotional questions assess your anxiety, frustration, and overall sense of handicap which you attribute to your hearing loss. You merely check or answer "Yes" if you experience difficulty in the situation described; "Sometimes" if you experience occasional difficulty in the given situation; or "No" if you rarely or never experience the problem. A score of "4" is awarded each Yes response, a score of "2" each Sometimes response, and a score of "0" for each No response. Points for each of the 10 items are added up and you can earn total scores which range from 0 to 40. The higher the number, the greater is the problem of hearing loss.

Table 6-I
Hearing Handicap Inventory for the Elderly—Screening [HHIE-S]

INSTRUCTIONS: The purpose of this questionnaire is to identify the problems your hearing loss may be causing you. Answer YES, SOMETIMES, or NO for each question. To obtain a total score, add up the "yes" (4 points), "sometimes" (2 points), and "no" (0 points) responses. If your score is greater than 10, a hearing test is recommended.

Yes	Sometimes	No
4	2	0

E1   Does a hearing problem cause you to feel embarrassed when you meet new people?

E2   Does a hearing problem cause you to feel frustrated when talking to members of your family?

S1   Do you have difficulty hearing when someone speaks in a whisper?

E3   Do you feel handicapped by a hearing problem?

S2   Does a hearing problem cause you difficulty when visiting friends, relatives or neighbors?

S3   Does a hearing problem cause you to attend religious services less often than you would like?

E4   Does a hearing problem cause you to have arguments with family members?

S4   Does a hearing problem cause you difficulty when listening to TV or radio?

E5   Do you feel that any difficulty with your hearing limits or hampers your personal or social life?

S5   Does a hearing problem cause you difficulty when in a restaurant with relatives or friends?

Table 6-II
Hearing Handicap Inventory for Adult—Screening [HHIA-S]

INSTRUCTIONS: The purpose of this questionnaire is to identify the problems your hearing loss may be causing you. Answer YES, SOMETIMES, or NO for each question. To obtain a total score, add up the "yes" (4 points), "sometimes" (2 points), and "no" (0 points) responses. If your score is greater than 10, a hearing test is recommended.

Yes	Sometimes	No
4	2	0

E1   Does a hearing problem cause you to feel embarrassed when you meet new people?

E2   Does a hearing problem cause you to feel frustrated when talking to members of your family?

S1   Do you have difficulty hearing/understanding co-workers, clients, customers?

E3   Do you feel handicapped by a hearing problem?

S2   Does a hearing problem cause you difficulty when visiting friends, relatives or neighbors?

S3   Does a hearing problem cause you difficulty in the movies or in the theater?

E4   Does a hearing problem cause you to have arguments with family members?

S4   Does a hearing problem cause you difficulty when listening to TV or radio?

E5   Do you feel that any difficulty with your hearing limits or hampers your personal or social life?

S5   Does a hearing problem cause you difficulty when in a restaurant with relatives or friends?

A score of 10 or greater signifies the necessity for referral to a hearing health care professional. More specifically, scores of 0-8 signify *no handicap;* scores of 10-22 signify *a mild to moderate handicap*; and scores of 24-40 suggest significant *self-perceived handicap.* As will be discussed in the next section, scores on the HHIE-S or HHIA-S are directly correlated to the purchase of a hearing aid and have been shown to improve after the initiation of hearing aid use. Finally, a companion version of each questionnaire is available for spouses or significant others to complete, enabling them to rate the extent of the problem posed by a hearing loss. The items, which are shown in Table 6-III, are comparable to those comprising the HHIE-S with the word "spouse (**SP**)" replacing "Your." The HHIE-SP is scored the same way as the original questionnaire. Interestingly, total scores often differ between you and your partner. In general, spousal ratings suggest a more significant handicap than you might perceive.

Candidacy for Hearing Aids

Recently, a number of investigators have demonstrated that desire to purchase hearing aids is directly linked to the score obtained on the HHIE-S or HHIA-S. Bess (1995) and his colleagues from Tennessee found that the extent of self-perceived hearing handicap on the 10-item screening version of the Hearing Handicap Inventory for the Elderly (HHIE-S) is predictive of hearing aid candidacy, in that it reliably distinguishes between people who ultimately purchase hearing aids and those who don't. Irrespective of the severity of hearing loss for pure tone signals (e.g. mild or moderate sensorineural hearing loss), persons in their study who actually purchased hearing aids were more handicapped as evidenced by higher scores on the HHIE-S, than those who did not. Thus, the investigators concluded that people who perceive themselves to be disabled or handicapped by a given hearing loss for pure tone signals are motivated to purchase hearing aids to reduce some of their communication difficulties.

A recent study reported by Kochkin (1996), who sampled many hearing aid owners and non-owners across the country, revealed that an individual's total score on one of the hearing handicap inventories (HHI) statistically predicted ownership of hearing aids. For example, 5.7 percent of survey respondents who scored a "0" on the HHI owned a hearing aid whereas 49 percent of those with a score of "28" owned hearing aids. In general, this study revealed that the average score on the HHI of non-hearing aid owners was 13.7 out of a total score of

Table 6-III
Hearing Handicap Inventory for the Elderly—Spouse [HHIE-SP]

INSTRUCTIONS: The purpose of this questionnaire is to identify the problems the hearing loss may be causing your spouse. Answer YES, SOMETIMES, or NO for each question. To obtain a total score, add up the "yes" (4 points), "sometimes" (2 points), and "no" (0 points) responses. If the score is greater than 10, a hearing test is recommended.

Yes	Sometimes	No
4	2	0

E1   Does a hearing problem cause your spouse to feel embarrassed when meeting new people?

E2   Does a hearing problem cause your spouse to feel frustrated when talking to members of your family?

S1   Does your spouse have difficulty hearing when someone speaks in a whisper?

E3   Does your spouse feel handicapped by a hearing problem?

S2   Does a hearing problem cause your spouse difficulty when visiting friends, relatives or neighbors?

S3   Does a hearing problem cause your spouse to attend religious services less often than he or she would like?

E4   Does a hearing problem cause your spouse to have arguments with family members?

S4   Does a hearing problem cause your spouse difficulty when listening to TV or radio?

E5   Do you feel that any difficulty with hearing limits or hampers your spouse's personal or social life?

S5   Does a hearing problem cause you difficulty when in a restaurant with relatives or friends?

40, compared to 20.8 percent for hearing aid owners. Interestingly, purchase of completely-in-the canal hearing aids is highly correlated to scores on the HHI as well. These studies demonstrate that self-perceived handicap, identified using a simple and easy screening tool, is linked to the decision on the part of individuals with hearing loss to purchase hearing aids. I encourage you to screen your hearing using one of the questionnaires included as Table 6-I or 6-II. If your total score adds up to 10 or more, you may consider scheduling a hearing test and learning about the options available so that you don't have to miss out on hearing.

The Impact of Hearing Loss

In general, hearing loss restricts one or more dimensions in the quality of life including communication function, mental status, emotional and social function. Specifically, hearing impairment has been shown to:

- negatively impact on communicative behavior
- alter psychosocial behavior
- strain family relations
- limit the enjoyment of daily activities
- jeopardize physical well-being
- interfere with the ability to live independently and safely
- potentially interfere with long distance contacts on the telephone
- jeopardize safety and security
- compromise efficiency at work
- interfere with one's ability to work with co-workers, and clients
- interfere with medical diagnosis, treatment and management
- interfere with compliance with pharmacologic regimens,
- and interfere with therapeutic interventions across all disciplines including social work, speech-language therapy, physical or occupational therapy.

An interesting aspect of hearing impairment which afflicts adults is the large variability in response to a given hearing loss. That is to say, two individuals with the same amount of hearing loss can react very differently and can experience different behavioral consequences. Accordingly, more and more audiologists include as part of a complete hearing assessment, questions about how a given hearing loss impacts on communication, social and emotional function. As will be demonstrated in the next section, despite some limitations in their ability to separate speech from noise, hearing aids have been shown to improve function in the areas you need assistance.

Your Readiness for Help

People with hearing problems typically seek out the assistance of a hearing health care provider when they finally realize that the hearing impairment is interfering with participation in and enjoyment of routine activities, and thus, is diminishing the quality of their lives. Hence, the decision about whether or not hearing aids are actually "worth the financial outlay," depends on if their actually reducing or eliminating the difficulties attributable to hearing loss. According to one source, the average time interval between an individual first noticing a hearing loss and seeking some form of evaluation and intervention is on the order of 10 years. It is hoped that the advent of smaller completely-in-the canal hearing aids, programmable and true digital hearing aids will lead to an earlier decision to reduce the consequences of hearing loss.

The typical trigger for seeking assistance is the person with mild to moderate hearing loss who realizes that the loss is interfering with enjoyment of routine activities, most notably television viewing and communicating with relatives and friends. The experience of Mrs. Girard, a 64-year-old woman, is a case in point. She had a moderate hearing loss which was most pronounced for high-pitched sounds such as /s/ or /sh/. She felt extremely frustrated because of difficulty understanding what others were saying when background noise was present (for example, in a restaurant or at a lecture). She first began having difficulty in small group situations, yet she was able to compensate so she didn't pay much attention to her problems. Within four to five years, her difficulties extended to large group situations, and finally she found that communicating in noisy environments posed a major problem for her. She finally decided to obtain a hearing assessment because, following her retirement, she chose to go back to school to earn a college degree, and the hearing loss was interfering with her ability to understand her instructors and fellow students. She had been to the theater and tried using an infrared system to help her understand. She was pleasantly surprised at how well she could understand the actors and actresses and decided to pursue the possibility of purchasing hearing aids.

Her provider recommended a programmable hearing aid system since this could be fine-tuned to help in situations Mrs. Girard found most troublesome. To help her decide if hearing aids were worth the money, she was advised to consider the extent to which hearing aids helped her in situations she found most problematic. For example, while amplified, was she having less difficulty understanding her fellow students, or understanding the instructor when attending a lecture in a large classroom? With hearing aids, was she feeling less frustrated in the above situations and less handicapped by her hearing loss? If she answered "Yes" or "Sometimes," then hearing aids were worth the investment. If not, she could have returned to her provider, explained her concerns, and the professional should have adjusted the devices, and counseled Mrs. Girard regarding what she should realistically expect from hearing aids. If after using the devices she continued to have reservations about whether hearing aids were helping in situations she considered important, then the devices may not have been the most appropriate to her needs, and alternative interventions should have been explored.

The bottom line for new users of hearing aids is, to what extent they are meeting or exceeding their expectations both socially and emotionally. It's incumbent on the provider to ensure that you have been instilled with realistic expectations, most notably that hearing aids cannot restore your hearing to normal, and that your most difficult listening situations may remain the most problematic, albeit less so, with hearing aids. Research conducted within the past five years has effectively demonstrated that hearing aids, in fact, reverse situational difficulties and emotional handicaps experienced by large numbers of individuals with acquired sensorineural hearing loss, yet some residual disability and handicap tends to remain.

Realistic Hearing Aid Performance and Benefits

In 1996 (Weinstein), I did a comprehensive review of studies on hearing aid benefit and satisfaction. It showed that hearing aids, either alone or in combination with three to six weeks of counseling-oriented audiological rehabilitation, can effectively reduce or minimize the disabilities and handicaps perceived by persons with adult onset sensorineural hearing loss. More specifically, in approximately four to five studies conducted across the country in a number of different settings including private practices, hospital clinics, and veterans administration centers, 70 to 80 percent of new hearing aid users experienced very dramatic reductions in the amount of their self-perceived hearing handicap. That is to say, for example, hearing impairments which were initially judged to be moderately to severely handicapping (60 percent on the HHI) improved to the point that new hearing aid users considered their hearing loss to be slightly or mildly handicapping (20 percent on the HHI) after only three weeks of hearing aid use.

When these new hearing aid users were recalled to the hearing clinics to ascertain how they were functioning with their hearing aids, in many of the studies, they derived significant benefit such that they perceived the hearing loss to be less handicapping socially and emotionally. This is depicted in Figure 6-1 which shows a graph of how percentage handicap, as judged by clients according to their responses to the HHI, changed (improved) from 60 percent before hearing aids were purchased to 20 percent after three weeks and one year of hearing aid use.

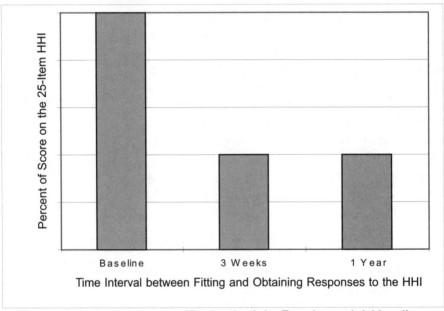

Figure 6-1: Improvement (Reduction) in Psychosocial Handicap according to Scores on HHI following One Year of Hearing Aid Use.

This represents a dramatic improvement and suggests that many of the problems people had when they came in for hearing aids—such as difficulty understanding friends, relatives, television and radio, or feeling upset by the hearing loss—were alleviated by hearing aid use. It's noteworthy that hearing aids did not "cure" all of each person's handicap. The reality of hearing aids is that they're helpful in a variety of situations, and can alleviate feelings of isolation. However, it's unrealistic to expect "a quick fix in all situations." Remember, expectations must be realistic so that you're not disappointed with hearing aid performance. A satisfied hearing aid user is one whose expectations match actual hearing aid performance.

There are times when new hearing aid users find they're not deriving the emotional and social benefits from hearing aids which had been expected. For example, take the case of a 55-year-old teacher who recently found out that he had a mild to moderate sensorineural hearing loss. He had reported some difficulty understanding speech, especially in a noisy classroom. His score on the Hearing Handicap Inventory (HHI) was 50 percent, suggesting that in fact he perceived his hearing loss as measured on the audiogram to be handicapping socially and emotionally. More particularly, he reported feeling handicapped, upset, embarrassed by and nervous from his inability to hear in a variety of situations, most notably at work (i.e. in the classroom), in movie theaters, and when socializing with friends and relatives. He decided to purchase binaural hearing aids to help him understand his students more easily. For a variety of reasons, behind-the-ear programmable instruments were recommended at the time of hearing aid selection. When he returned to his provider for his three-week follow-up appointment to determine how he was functioning with his hearing aids, he indicated that it was not helpful in the situations that mattered. His score on the HHI verified that the hearing aids, in fact, were not helping him, as the score remained at 50 percent, suggesting absolutely no benefit.

The hearing care professional made some modifications to the hearing aids, and the quality of the amplified signal improved. However, he remained opposed to continuing. The provider then suggested that the client try in-the-ear hearing aids having similar electroacoustic features. This version was a new model having been recently introduced by the hearing aid company. He agreed to try them, was instructed on how to use them, was counseled regarding expected benefits, and returned three weeks later for a follow-up visit. To his relief and the provider's amazement, the client was quite pleased with the hearing aids, indicating that they were helping him in situations which were important to him and were alleviating some of the negative emotions attributable to his hearing loss. Thereby, he felt less handicapped, anxious, and upset.

Responses to the HHIE confirmed his subjective reports as his total score improved to 10 percent suggesting a minimal hearing handicap with his new in-the-ear hearing aids. He continued to receive benefit after six months of hearing aid use. The pattern of findings is depicted in Figure 6-2. This case highlights the value of feedback from you, the client, and the importance of objectively quantifying performance with a given hearing aid. Responses to a questionnaire, such as the HHI, can assist you in recognizing if and in what situations hearing aids are helping.

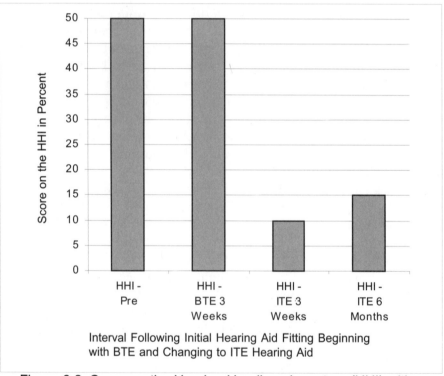

Figure 6-2: Score on the Hearing Handicap Inventory (HHI) with a behind-the-ear (BTE) and an in-the-ear (ITE) hearing aid at varying time intervals following the initial hearing aid fitting.

Another interesting way in which responses to the HHI can be helpful to both the new hearing aid user and the provider is when a hearing aid seems helpful but its value does not justify the expense. A retired attorney noted that now that he was no longer confined to an office or a courtroom, he was having difficulty functioning in the variety of new situations in which he found himself. He participated in a hearing screening at a local health fair and found out he was unable to hear pure tones being presented and scored an 18 on the screening version of the Hearing Handicap Inventory. The audiologist provided a referral to a hearing health care professional who urged him to obtain a complete hearing test. He scheduled an appointment with a provider and underwent a series of pure tone and speech tests to determine the extent of hearing loss. Results revealed a mild to moderate high frequency sensorineural hearing loss in each ear, consistent with the type of hearing loss attributable to the aging process. The score on the 25-item Hearing Handicap Inventory suggested a moderate psychosocial handicap (score of 40 percent). In light of the clients complaints, the configuration of hearing loss (high frequency), and its severity (mild to moderate), binaural completely-in-the canal hearing aids were recommended. The client was instructed to return to the provider after three weeks of hearing aid use to verify the response and to monitor his performance with them.

Interestingly, on the return visit, the client complained that the hearing aids were amplifying too much noise, and were not helpful in situations he considered most important (namely small groups) where background noise was present. The HHI score of 38 percent verified that in fact the hearing aids were not providing him with much assistance. After modification, the client left expressing satisfaction. Upon the return visit (three weeks later, six weeks from the initial fitting), the client reported that the hearing aids were helping him to function well and enjoy numerous leisure activities in which he was participating. The HHI score at this time improved some 30 points to 8 percent, suggesting a minimal psychosocial handicap attributable to the hearing loss. Once again, objective verification for the client was helpful, enabling him to justify the expenditure.

There are occasions when individuals who were previously functioning well with their hearing aids can experience a decline in performance. Take for example the case of Mr. Osborn, an 80-year-old accountant who continues to work part-time. He had worn behind-the-ear hearing aids for 10 years and up until recently was quite satisfied with them. They were helping to alleviate speech understanding difficulties attributable to his bilateral, moderate, sensorineural hearing loss, which he first noted on his 65th birthday.

Pure tone test results at his most recent examination by his provider revealed that his hearing had remained the same (moderate in degree). However, his speech understanding problems had declined dramatically, especially in noisy situations. A complete audiological work-up revealed a central auditory processing problem which can accompany the aging process.* Interestingly, the pattern of findings on the HHI confirmed Mr. Osborn's subjective complaints in that he no longer was benefiting from the hearing aids. As is evident from Figure 6-3, the initial HHI score was 50 percent (prior to hearing aids), improving to 24 percent after the initial hearing aid fitting. His HHI score was between 24 percent and 30 percent over time, suggesting considerable reduction (improvement) in psychosocial handicap attributable to hearing aid use.

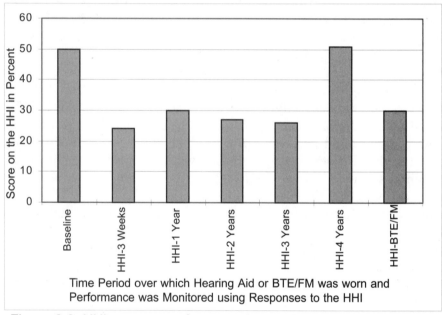

Figure 6-3: HHI scores over four-year time period with hearing aid and BTE/FM device.

Four years later, at Mr. Osborn's most recent visit, the HHI score returned to 52 percent, confirming limited hearing aid benefit. His

---

* **This problem implies that the ability to understand speech is most difficult in sub-optimal listening environments (e.g. noise, reverberation), and that the difficulties are much greater than one would expect from the pattern of pure tone hearing loss.**

provider recommended a conventional behind-the-ear aid with an FM receiver incorporated into the hearing aid case. The advantage of an FM system is the improved signal-to-noise ratio achieved by bringing the microphone closer to the source of sound. Essentially, FM systems bridge the acoustical space between the sound source and the listener by eliminating the detrimental effects on speech understanding: distance, noise and reverberation. The primary advantages of a BTE/FM system are that it can be used as a regular hearing aid, or as an FM receiver bringing the signal directly to the user's ear, or as both an FM system and a hearing aid. It's ideal when driving in a car, when conversing in a noisy environment, and when at a lecture or in a restaurant. Mr. Osborn, at the urging of his wife, agreed to give the BTE/FM system a try and was immediately impressed with the clarity of the signal, especially when he was tested with noise present in the background. Mr. and Mrs. Osborn were counseled on how to use the hearing aid and upon their return visit were happy to report that speech understanding in the most difficult situations had improved dramatically. The HHI score of 28 percent verified that Mr. Osborn was deriving substantial benefit from the new device. Figure 6-3 summarizes the pattern of HHI scores over time with the hearing aids and with the BTE/FM system.

As health care systems evolve, and managed care agencies play an increasingly important role in the delivery of services, it is incumbent upon you to obtain information which can help you appreciate the value of your hearing aids. This information can help justify what might appear as the high cost of present-day hearing aids. It's clear that hearing aids do provide quality of life benefits. Your needs and expectations can be realized when hearing care professionals listen to you the consumer, either by modifying the response of a hearing aid, substituting one style hearing aid for another, or replacing a conventional hearing aid with an assistive listening device to ensure adequate benefit.

A Final Word

To gain full benefit from hearing aids, you must be informed, have realistic expectations and patience, and you must purchase your hearing aids from a professional with whom you have confidence and rapport. It's also of utmost importance to have a firm idea about what you want from hearing aids. These are your self-perceptions. Completion of a self-report questionnaire prior to and after purchasing hearing aids can help you match perceptions of what you want hearing aids to do for you, against your expectations as established by your hearing health care professional. The closer this match, the more satisfied you'll be with your hearing aids. Consider the self-report questionnaire as a checklist against which you can judge the extent to which your needs are being met.

References

Bess, F. Applications of the hearing handicap inventory for the elderly—screening version (HHIE-S). The Hearing Journal, Vol. 48, 51-57, 1995.

Kochkin, S. MarkeTrak IV: 10-year trends in the hearing aid market—has anything changed? The Hearing Journal, Vol. 49, 23-33, 1996.

Ross, M. You've done something about it! Helpful hints to the new hearing aid user. SHHH Journal, Vol. 17, 7-11, 1996.

Self Help for Hard of Hearing People, Inc. Position statement on group hearing aid orientation programs. SHHH Journal, Vol. 17, 29, 1996.

Weinstein, B. Treatment efficacy: hearing aids in the management of hearing loss in adults. Journal Speech and Hearing Research. Vol. 39, S37-S45, 1996.

CHAPTER SEVEN

Hearing Aid Technology

Robert W. Sweetow, Ph.D.

Dr. Sweetow is Director of Audiology and Clinical Professor in the Department of Otolaryngology at the Medical Center of the University of California, San Francisco. He received his Ph.D. from Northwestern University in 1977. He holds a Master of Arts degree from the University of Southern California and a Bachelor of Science degree from the University of Iowa. Dr. Sweetow has lectured worldwide, and has authored numerous textbook chapters and over 60 scientific articles on tinnitus and amplification for the hearing impaired. In addition to his major interest in sports, he's been attempting to relax as a fisherman, and is still looking for that "Big One" that got away.

There are many myths and misconceptions regarding hearing aids. The objective of this chapter is to prepare you, the consumer, with accurate up-to-date information to help in your decision to upgrade or try new hearing aids. As technology advances, and as social and workplace demands change, so do the criteria for candidacy for wearable amplification. Thirty years ago, many hearing health care professionals believed that only people with conductive hearing loss could be helped by hearing aids. Patients were often told that hearing aids could make sounds *louder*, (just like turning up the volume on a radio), but would not necessarily make sounds *clearer*. This thinking was reinforced by reports of unfavorable results from those hearing impaired patients who did try hearing aids and who still couldn't understand speech clearly, particularly in noisy places.

Of course, it's now recognized that early attempts at fitting sensorineural impaired listeners with hearing aids were seriously hindered by the limited sound quality produced by these early devices; by the limited choice of electronic variations; and by poor fitting strategies used in trying to determine the best manner to amplify speech without making it too loud or too noisy.

In the early days of fitting hearing aids, professionals often tried to determine who was a candidate on the basis of the degree of hearing loss shown on the hearing test. You remember that when your hearing was tested, the audiologist or hearing instrument specialist used beeping tones and made the sounds louder and softer until you could no longer hear them. As described in Chapter 4, the point at which you could just barely hear a sound is called your threshold. These sounds are measured in decibels (dB). Classifications used two decades ago stated that hearing better than 25 dB was normal; 26-50 dB was a mild loss; 51-70 dB was a moderate loss; 71-90 dB was a severe loss; and 91 dB and poorer was a profound loss. Strict application of these categories isn't adequate to describe the impact hearing loss has on your life. Indeed, it oversimplifies the complexities of hearing impairment. Today, we realize that *properly fitted hearing aids can provide benefit even if you have a relatively mild hearing loss*.

In addition to the previous belief among physicians and some hearing professionals that you couldn't successfully use hearing aids if you had nerve damage, it was also thought that you couldn't use hearing aids if you had normal hearing for low-pitched sounds (up to 1500 or 2000 Hz); or if you had a hearing loss in only one ear, or if your speech understanding abilities were reduced, and/or if you have difficulty tolerating loud sounds, for example, a crying baby. Advances in technology now allow for good fittings for most of these patients.

Present-Day Candidacy For Hearing Aids

In the past several years, hearing aid technology has advanced to the point where the question of candidacy is now based more on your communicative *needs* rather than purely on the test results obtained in a soundproof room. That is, your own personal, *subjective needs*. A good litmus test is to ask yourself whether you feel stressed or fatigued after a day of straining to hear. Hearing aids may simply relieve this strain, rather than making sounds louder or allowing you to understand all speech in all listening environments. Reducing strain alone can be a very significant benefit, not only to you, but to those trying to talk to you. Thus, it's often advisable to go through a trial period to determine whether benefit warrants the expense.

Occupational and social demands vary greatly among individuals. A judge who has a mild hearing loss may desperately need amplification, while a retired elderly patient living alone who has the exact same degree of hearing loss may not. You must unselfishly examine whether you're becoming a burden to others, even if you do not personally recognize difficulty hearing. *Remember that wearing a hearing aid may be a mark of courtesy to others*. Unfortunately, despite the need, you, like many patients, may resist trying hearing aids. Two common factors characterizing the response in people who have been told they should wear amplification are that practically no one wants to wear hearing aids, and no one wants to spend money or waste time solving a problem unless they perceive that a problem exists and a solution is readily attainable. Opposition to wearing hearing aids usually stems from three main reasons.

First is *hearsay*. Most everyone has friends or relatives who have purchased hearing aids currently residing in their dresser drawers. These unsuccessful wearers of amplification are more than happy to spread the gospel on the limitations (some accurate, some not) of hearing aids. Often, these unsuccessful experiences occurred in extremely difficult listening environments in which even people with normal hearing had trouble understanding speech. Second, despite the fact that people of all ages have hearing impairment and use amplification, there's an undeniable *social stigma* attached to wearing hearing aids. The problem of vanity has been eased, in part, by the continuing trend toward miniaturization of hearing devices. However, not all hearing impaired listeners are candidates for the very tiny new hearing aids. Thus, stigma is likely to remain a difficult hurdle to overcome. The third main reason for opposition to hearing aid use is the perception that the relatively high cost of hearing aids is not reflected in the value and benefits they provide. When making a decision as to whether this is the right time for you to try hearing aids, you must weigh whether the financial investment can be offset by the improvement in life you might achieve by reducing your hearing difficulty. Be sure to consider improvements from a social, emotional, and occupational perspective, also considering activities you would like to undertake but have given up because of communication difficulties.

It's a double-edged sword when it comes to dispensing hearing aids to a person who's not motivated to wear amplification. On one hand, a poorly motivated patient is not the best candidate for amplification regardless of the degree of hearing loss. So, from this perspective, the answer to the question of whether a steadfastly reluctant patient should be forced into trying a hearing aid is probably *no*. It may be difficult to undo the damage that may be done if the borderline candidate prematurely tries, and fails with amplification. If you feel you're absolutely opposed to trying hearing aids at this time, and if you're convinced you'll fail, it may be advisable to wait until another time when you may more clearly perceive the need. On the other hand, keep in mind that it's possible you may be pleasantly surprised. Remember that, as discussed later in this chapter, there have been more changes in hearing aids during the last five years than in the previous thirty.

Hearing Aid Styles

In the early 1950s, you would have been limited to a choice of two styles of hearing instruments: body borne or in-eyeglass frames. Neither of these styles are in common use in the U.S. today, yet still remain popular in third world countries. Currently, you have a great number of options regarding hearing aid style (See Figure 7-1). Behind-the-ear (BTE) hearing aids sit over the outer ear and are connected to an earmold located in the concha (bowl) of the ear and ear canal. There are a variety of sizes, shapes, and models of hearing aids which fit within a plastic shell and are worn entirely inside the ear. They include the custom in-the-ear (ITE) model (which may completely fill, or occlude, the bowl and ear canal), the thinner low profile, the partially occluding half concha, the even less occluding helix model for high frequency losses, the in-the-canal (ITC), and the tiniest of styles, the completely-in-canal (CIC) hearing aids.

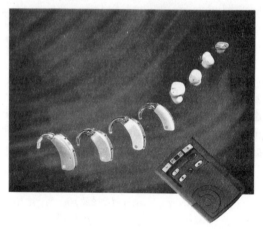

Figure 7-1: Range of hearing aid styles from (left to right) behind-the-ear to completely-in-the-canal.

I strongly discourage you from selecting the style of hearing aids you're going to try strictly on the basis of cosmetic factors. While cosmetic considerations may be important, the decision as to which style hearing aids are most appropriate for you should be based on both physical as well as audiological factors.

Physical factors

Anatomical characteristics may dictate the style; for example, behind-the-ear hearing aids may not be able to be used if you have deformed outer ears; the depth of your concha may determine the appropriateness of certain in-the-ear model instruments; and in order to be able to wear the in-the-canal or the completely-in-canal types of hearing aids, your ear canal must be of sufficient diameter and must have a sharp enough bend to retain the aid, but not be so curvy that it prevents easy insertion and removal.

Manual dexterity is essential to handling some of the smaller style hearing aids. Not only is removal and insertion of canal hearing aids difficult for certain people, particularly some older folks, but the ability to manipulate the volume control and battery must be considered and assessed before you decide that a certain style is right for you. Also, some people need hearing aids which are large enough to accommodate a vent (hole) drilled into it, allowing air to enter the ear canal. Without this ventilation, you may perceive a "plugged up" feeling or you may sound to yourself that you're "in a barrel" when you speak. This phenomenon is commonly referred to as the "occlusion effect." In addition, if your ears produce excessive cerumen (earwax), you may be better off by not wearing canal, or even certain full ITE hearing aids.

Medical Contraindications such as draining ears or other medical problems may prevent the use of any hearing aid apparatus blocking your ear canals. In this instance, you'll need open, non-occluding earmolds or possibly bone conduction-type systems. These types of hearing aids are beyond the scope of this discussion, and can be reviewed by your hearing health care provider if they're applicable to you.

Audiological factors:

The audiometric configuration on your audiogram may show certain frequencies (pitches) which have normal hearing. For example, in the low frequencies, you may be best served by systems that don't occlude (block) your ear canal.

The degree of loss may predict the need for a specific kind of hearing aid. For example, severe and profound hearing losses are best served by BTE-style hearing aids.

Special features may be indicated, such as directional microphones (which primarily amplify signals emanating from in front of you) and/or the addition of a telecoil (a magnetic induction loop). Telecoils allow sound to bypass the hearing aid microphone and amplify signals received electromagnetically (when used with telephone handsets designed for such use). In addition to allowing a hearing aid user to listen to telephone signals without getting feedback (whistling), telecoils interface with a variety of assistive listening devices.

Acoustic feedback refers to that whistling or ringing sound often produced when you cup your hand over your ear while wearing a hearing aid. It also occurs when the hearing aid is not properly or snugly inserted in your ear. Before discussing feedback, it would help to first describe the basic components that are found in all hearing aids. Figure 7-2 shows the series of events that occur in a typical hearing aid: First, sound enters into a <u>microphone</u>. Next, this sound is transformed into an electrical current as the diaphragm of the microphone moves back and forth. Then, the electrical current is fed into an <u>amplifier</u> and filtered by electrical components that establish how much relative amplification will be provided for the different frequencies. For example, most hearing aids try to amplify the high pitches more than the low pitches. The overall amount of amplification is governed by a <u>volume control.</u> The newly formed amplified electrical signal is then fed to a <u>receiver</u>, also called a loudspeaker. The receiver turns the electrical signal back into sound waves which exit the hearing aid and enter the ear canal through the <u>earmold</u> for BTE hearing aids, or a tube in the plastic shell for custom styles. Also, all hearing aids are run by a tiny <u>battery</u>, which generally lasts for between one to three weeks.

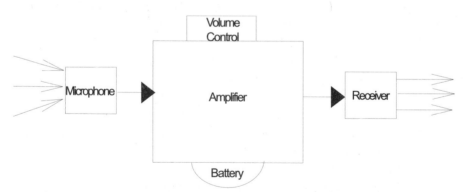

FIGURE 7-2: Transmission of Sound Through a Hearing Aid

Generally speaking, the closer the microphone is to the exit point of the amplified sound from the hearing aid or earmold, the greater the likelihood of feedback. This occurs when amplified sound from the earmold leaks back into the hearing aid's microphone and is re-amplified. This is a very important consideration in the selection and fitting of amplification. BTE hearing aids often have an advantage over smaller ITE or ITC styles in this regard since there's more physical distance between the microphone and the receiver. Many manufacturers provide "feedback controls" which are adjustments that reduce high frequency amplification. While this does indeed accomplish the desired effect of reducing feedback, it may do so at the expense of also reducing the audibility of the vitally important high frequency consonant sounds which are essential for understanding speech. Therefore, this approach to feedback control is often not an acceptable trade-off. The best solution is to make sure that the earmold or plastic shell fits perfectly in the ear. This is why it's important that your hearing health care professional takes a good impression of your ears before you obtain hearing aids. If you haven't yet had an earmold impression taken, don't worry. It doesn't hurt. Your provider will first place a cotton or foam block in your ear canal and will then inject liquid material in your ear which will harden in about five minutes. It's a similar process to getting impressions made by the dentist, except you don't need Novocain!

Small Hearing Aids

If you're like most patients, perhaps one of the first questions you have is whether you can use one of the really small, "invisible" hearing aids (the ITC or CIC styles). Hearing aids keep getting smaller but small does not necessarily mean better. A canal-style hearing aid implies that no part of the hearing aid extends into the concha (bowl) area. There are two types: the ITC aid fills the outer half, or soft, cartilaginous portion of the ear canal while the CIC is inserted deeper in the ear canal and extends into the inner half. The CIC hearing aid is so tiny that it must be removed from the ear by pulling on a monofilament extension cord that rests at the bottom of the concha.

Advantages **Of Canal Hearing Aids:**
1) They are the most *"invisible"* systems available.
2) The microphone lies either within, or at the entrance of the ear canal and thus is able to benefit fully from the *natural amplification* of the outer ear bowl.
3) The receiver of the hearing aid is located closer to the eardrum, where the amount of air trapped in the ear canal that needs to vibrate is less than for most other fittings. Therefore, *less hearing aid amplification is needed* to produce the same sound pressure

at the eardrum. This often results in lower distortion levels and less likelihood of acoustic feedback.

Disadvantages of ITC or CIC fittings:

1) If the receiver stops in the outer half of the canal, it may be *subject to breakdowns* due to blockage from earwax.
2) If the receiver terminates in the outer, cartilaginous portion of the canal, you may notice the "occlusion" or "barrel effect" in which your <u>own voice sounds hollow</u> as if you were in a tunnel. You can demonstrate this effect even without a hearing aid by humming after you occlude your ear canal with your finger, then comparing the sound of your own voice when your canal is open.
3) If the receiver stops in the inner, bony portion of the canal, this deeper canal placement may be <u>physically uncomfortable</u> to you because the skin is much thinner than it is at the outer part of the canal.
4) Because the aid is so small, <u>there may not be adequate room to vent</u> the aid in order to relieve pressure build-up or to release unwanted low frequency amplification.
5) They are <u>not powerful enough to fit severe or profound losses</u>.
6) Adequate manual <u>dexterity is essential</u>.

It's not unusual to find that the most important factors determining success or failure of a fitting are those unrelated to audiometric findings. In particular, you must take into consideration all of the following: your age and general physical and mental health; your motivation (as opposed to that of your family's); finances; cosmetic considerations; and your communication needs. It's heartening to note that the primary reasons for rejection of hearing aids, after people try them, are less related to finances and cosmetics than they are to difficulty hearing in background noise, and discomfort from loud sounds. These problems are well on the way to being lessened by modern day hearing aids and fitting techniques.

One Versus Two Hearing Aids

You may be wondering whether it's necessary for you to wear two hearing aids (binaural) as opposed to one (monaural). Financial or psychological (including vanity) considerations may be entering your mind. Over 60 percent of hearing aid fittings in the United States are binaural. There are a variety of reasons why binaural hearing is better than monaural. Of these, perhaps the most important are:

Hearing Better in Noise

You may be better able to detect sounds immersed in background noise if the signals reaching each ear are slightly different. When the brain receives different, yet audible signals at the two ears, it has the ability to compare and contrast the primary signal (speech) from the secondary signal (noise), better than if the signal is received monaurally.

Optimizing Your Position

Because most acoustic environments have fluctuating background noise, it's likely you'll find yourself in adverse positions (where the "good" ear may be closer to the unwanted background noise and the "bad" ear is closer to desired sound source, i.e. speech) nearly 50 percent of the time. When sound crosses your head and body, there's a decrease of intensity (loudness) that is greater for high frequencies—those most responsible for comprehending consonant sounds, than for the low frequencies. Thus, if you wear only one hearing aid, and if the person you want to hear is sitting on your unaided side while sounds of dishes clattering are near the ear in which the hearing aid is worn, noise will be amplified by the hearing aid (while speech loses power as it crosses your head and body). Obviously, this places you at a great disadvantage. On the other hand, if hearing aids are worn in both ears, this situation is much less likely to occur because each ear would receive amplification compensating for the loss of power resulting from the speech "crossing" the head.

Improving Localization Ability

We humans are able to determine from where a sound is coming by means of: (a) differences in relative loudness between the ears; (b) differences in the relative time of arrival of sound at the two ears; and (c) differences in the frequency (or pitch) of the signal at the two ears. Your brain performs these analyses without any conscious effort. The ability of your brain to utilize such subtleties, however, is dependent on the differences being audible in both ears. If what you want to hear is heard in only one ear, your brain cannot take advantage of these cues.

Possibility of Deterioration in the Unaided Ear

Remember that although your ear is the organ that receives sound, it's your brain that ultimately "hears" it. Some researchers believe that if you have two similarly impaired ears, and you wear monaural amplification, you may show more rapid deterioration in the unaided ear than you would if you wore hearing aids in both ears. It's debatable whether lesser usage of an ear really produces physical changes in that ear. However, there is ample evidence of neurological degeneration that occurs due to lack of stimulation.

Combining Binaural Signals

A very soft sound can be heard at lower levels when two ears are in operation rather than one. Similarly, a loud sound is perceived as being less uncomfortable when two ears hear it. So, you can achieve the same loudness perception from binaural hearing aids which are set at lower volume than you could with only one aid. By using a lower volume setting, you reduce the likelihood of feedback and distortion problems. Therefore, the general rule is that unless you have a significant difference (asymmetry) between your ears, you should consider a trial with two hearing aids, rather than one. If during the trial you really believe you are better off with just one hearing aid, you can usually return the other one.

Some ears simply cannot use a hearing aid. For example, perhaps your ear cannot be blocked because it drains, or it has had certain surgeries, or it's completely deaf, or unable to understand speech (even when it's loud enough), or it cannot tolerate loud sounds. If this is the case, your hearing health care professional can prescribe special types of hearing aids that partially compensate for the lack of binaural listening by routing the amplified signal from one side of the head to the other. These hearing aids are called CROS (Contralateral Routing of the Signal). There are a number of variations of this type of hearing aid system that can be tailored to your needs.

The Evolution of Hearing Aids

There are two basic rules that must be followed if a hearing aid fitting is to be successful: soft sounds must be made audible; and loud sounds must not be uncomfortable. The reason is that if you have a sensorineual hearing loss, your hearing loss is for soft sounds but not for loud sounds. Therefore, hearing aids have changed over the past three decades in the following ways.

1. Linear Hearing Aids

In the past, many users reported that in order to hear soft sounds, they had to turn their hearing aids up quite loud. This did indeed allow them to hear soft sounds but it also produced the undesirable effect of making loud sounds uncomfortable. Here's why.

Imagine that a certain level of sound enters the hearing aid, let's say 65 dB (which happens to be about the level of normal conversational speech). To make this speech comfortable, the volume of the hearing aid might be set so that it produces 25 dB of amplification. Therefore, 90 dB comes into the ear canal (65 plus 25). Now, lets imagine that the sound coming into the hearing aid suddenly becomes much louder, as might occur in a restaurant when people at your table start to laugh at a joke. If you are wearing a conventional hearing aid, the sound coming into it is now increased to 90 dB, and this type of hearing aid will still add 25 dB of amplification, so the sound in your ear canal actually becomes 115 dB. For most people, this will be entirely too loud and uncomfortable, and your reaction will be to try and turn it down using the volume control. This is why you'll see most people with conventional hearing aids turn the volume control quite often when the sound intensity in the surrounding environment changes. Hearing aids which produce the same amount of amplification regardless of the loudness of the sound entering are technically categorized as *linear, one channel, conventional* hearing aids.

2. Non-Linear, *Single Channel*

A few years ago a new type of hearing aid was introduced using more advanced technology called non-linear, or compression. With this system, there's more amplification given to soft sounds than there is for louder sounds. In other words, when sounds are above a certain level set in the hearing aid, it's as if an invisible finger reaches up and automatically moves the volume down for you, and vice versa, when the sound environment becomes lower than a certain level. This type of non-linear hearing aid basically squeezes a wide range of loudness into a narrower range, which has generated the other descriptive name of *compression hearing aids*. Going back to the earlier example, now with the non-linear type, when sounds entering the hearing aid suddenly increase to 90 dB, the amplification is lowered from 25 dB to 10 dB. Therefore, the sound reaching your eardrum is a more comfortable 100 dB as opposed to the uncomfortable 115.

3. Non-Linear, *Multichannel*

While non-linear one channel hearing aids help restore loudness perception to you, one major weakness remains: Your loudness growth pattern may be different from one pitch to another. That is, you might find high-pitched sounds (dishes clanging) seem painfully loud to you but low-pitched sounds (a refrigerator humming) do not. Therefore, the amount of compression may need to be different for various frequencies. This is where the next step up in circuitry sophistication comes in, *non-linear multiple channel*.

With multiple channels, compression characteristics of the hearing aid will be tailored to your personal needs based upon how loud you interpret certain sounds to be for various frequencies. Perhaps there will be a lot of compression for the high frequencies but very little for the low frequencies. This feature helps to make sounds appear comfortably loud for you. The second thing multiple compression accomplishes may be even more important. If your hearing aid system has only one channel, a loud noise made up of mostly low frequencies, (as might be found in cocktail parties) would tell the hearing aid that it needs to lower its amplification for all frequencies. This would help to keep the sound from being too loud, but it would make some of the high frequency sounds (like consonants) too soft to hear.

A multiple channel hearing aid, on the other hand, in that same loud, low frequency noise situation, would decrease the amplification for low frequencies, making sound comfortable without changing the amplification for the high frequencies (thus preserving audibility of important high frequency consonant sounds). This system can actually produce additional high frequency amplification while simultaneously reducing low frequency amplification, all depending on the sound environment.

Non-linear, multiple channel hearing aids act not only as a means of loudness control, but also as a means of differentiating the amount of amplification given to different parts of the speech signal. If fitted correctly, they can dampen the strong elements of speech, such as vowels, and enhance the delicate speech elements such as the /s/, /sh/ and /f/ sounds. This will greatly improve speech clarity, especially in difficult listening environments.

4. Multiple Programs versus Automatic

Some people find it useful to be able to change hearing aid characteristics depending on the environment they are in. Of course, you can't keep running back to your provider each time you enter a new environment. Another option would be to have hearing aids that have several programs that you can easily select simply by touching a button located on the hearing aid or on a separate remote control. For example, one button could select a hearing aid program which is best suited to listening to one person, another program to listening in a restaurant, while yet another for music. This can also be useful if you have a fluctuating hearing loss.

Many modern hearing aids are automatic in the way they regulate volume. Often, these hearing aids regulate themselves so automatically that they don't contain a volume control. You may find this to your liking if you're the type who doesn't like to frequently adjust your hearing aids, or, you may feel that not having a volume control takes away too much control from you. This is something you should discuss carefully with your hearing health care provider.

5. Digitally-Programmable Hearing Aids

Hearing aids that are programmed, or set, by your hearing health care provider, via an external computer, or computer-like instrument are called *digitally programmable*. Not all hearing impaired listeners require the use of these programmable hearing aids. Furthermore, programmability, per se, does not always imply superior listening performance. The basic advantage of programmable is the flexibility for your hearing care professional to change the programs in the hearing aids as your needs may change. Often, preferences for sound amplification changes over time after you have used the hearing aids for awhile. For instance, if you're a new user, you may not want hearing aids to amplify high pitches too much because they might seem too sharp or tinny. But after you've grown accustomed to hearing sounds you may not have heard for a long time, you may want to hear some of these high-pitched sounds. With a programmable system, your hearing health care provider can alter the amplification in your instruments by boosting higher pitches.

6. Digital Hearing Aids

All the hearing aids mentioned so far have been electronic devices of the conventional analog class. The latest advance in hearing aids is the introduction of fully digital. A digital hearing aid has a computer chip within doing the amplifier work instead of the traditional analog circuitry. It's actually a miniature computer in itself. This is a major breakthrough in technology because it greatly increases the amount of sound processing possible in the given amount of space.

The potential improvement from digital hearing aids is exciting and far-reaching because they have minimal distortion, giving some a clearer, crisper quality. The first commercially available digital hearing aids have taken all the benefits from the advanced non-linear multichannel hearing aids and improved them even further. This means they have the ability to analyze the sound environment and adapt the amplification accordingly, enhancing speech clarity. This is all done automatically without the need for volume or remote controls.

In the future, we can expect more and more intelligence built into digital systems as research comes up with newer and more advanced compensation strategies. It's even possible that one day all hearing instruments may be digital.

The Disadvantages of Programmable and Digital Hearing Aids

1) The initial investment tends to be higher than non-programmable, analog hearing aids.
2) Not all hearing care professionals have the equipment, training, and knowledge to work with these more advanced systems.
3) Some programmable systems require that you carry a remote control, typically the size of a pen or pocket calculator. Some people find this to be an unpleasant burden, while others like the idea of being able to control volume levels.

Determining the Proper Selection for You

Given the recent improvements in hearing aids and the number of available options, it's helpful to consider how hearing aid selection procedures have changed. In the past, providers often decided which was the "best" system for an individual by comparing which of two or three hearing aids produced the highest word recognition score. This score was obtained by having you listen and then repeat single syllable words (such as "dog," or "house"). It is now acknowledged that this comparative approach was flawed in a number of respects. For example, single syllable words presented in a quiet, non-reverberant environment are not representative of the real world. Furthermore, it's now believed that a period of time is needed to adjust, or acclimate, to various amplification systems. Perhaps most important, however, is the current thinking concerning the importance of restoring normal loudness relations, as just discussed. The comparative approach largely ignored this factor.

Currently, many hearing aid selection procedures use computers. The computer takes into account your hearing test results, your ability to tolerate loud sounds, and the types of environments you encounter most of the time. Based on this information, the computer tells your hearing health care provider which models may be appropriate for you, and which settings would best serve your needs. These suggestions, however, are only a jumping-off place. Fine-tuning adjustments are then made based on your individual preferences. The appropriateness of the fitting may then be verified by having you listen to and repeat words presented in quiet or background noise. It's also useful to verify the fitting by measuring the sound produced by the hearing aid right in your ear. This is done using a tiny microphone placed inside your ear canal and connected to specialized computer equipment. Not all providers use this equipment, but many find it extremely useful both for troubleshooting complaints and for ensuring that the expected amount of amplified sound is reaching your eardrum.

The Limitations Of Hearing Aids

Hearing aids are meant to minimize listening fatigue and to improve ease of communication. Thus, they're not meant to allow you to "hear a pin drop," and there are going to be circumstances in which hearing aids don't give you all the benefits you'd like. The most frequent complaints voiced by hearing aid users are that noise is amplified too much, certain sounds become too loud to bear, and some speech remains unclear.

Despite marketing claims, there are no hearing aids that effectively eliminate background noise. If all the sound energy that make up noise were eliminated, important segments of speech would also be missing. Also, remember that normal listeners experience background noise daily. If all background noise were eliminated, the acoustic world would be quite boring and unnatural. Even so, don't hesitate to discuss your perception of background noise with your provider so that your hearing aids can be fine-tuned to reach the best compromise.

With regard to clarity, remember that hearing aids are *aids* to hearing. They are not new ears, and they cannot correct for certain limitations in understanding that are more related to brain functioning than to hearing.

You may find that your own voice sounds odd when wearing hearing aids. The reason this occurs is that when you speak, you produce low frequency vibrations in your ear canals. When you're unaided, your ears are open, allowing these vibrations to escape from your ear canals out into the air. As touched on earlier, if your ears are blocked, these low frequency sounds are trapped in your ear canals and cannot escape. This increase in low frequency perception might make you sound as if you were talking in a barrel or experiencing an echo. This "occlusion effect" can be minimized by: 1) keeping the ear as open as possible, perhaps by means of vents (holes) drilled into the earmold or plastic shell; 2) reducing low frequency amplification; 3) using an earmold or ITE shell that sits deeply, reaching the inner half of the canal, thus reducing vibration; 4) or conversely, having the canal portion of the shell not set so deeply in the ear.

As mentioned earlier, a common annoyance is the presence of feedback. It doesn't mean that the hearing aid is malfunctioning. There are two types of acoustic feedback: that produced internally from the hearing aid indicating its need for repair, and the more common external feedback produced by a leakage of amplified sound out of the ear canal and back into the microphone of the hearing aid. Usually, external feedback can be corrected by 1) re-positioning or possibly remaking the earmold or the plastic shell; 2) plugging, or reducing the diameter of any vents; or 3) reducing the amount of high frequency amplification, which is usually an unacceptable trade-off because of the resultant loss of high frequency consonant audibility.

Another common limitation of hearing aids is that you may have more difficulty hearing when the sound source is at a distance from you. This occurs, for example, in large conference rooms or auditoriums. Loudness (intensity) decreases as physical distance increases. Unfortunately, most background noise surrounds you, so while the intensity of speech decreases with distance, the intensity of noise may not. This is one reason why hearing aids effectively transmit sound if the speaker talks right into the microphone, but at longer, more realistic distances, reception diminishes. It would be ideal if sound produced at the source transferred directly to you without losing any intensity. It's obviously impractical, however, to ask someone speaking to you to constantly move closer to your ear.

One way of achieving this effect is by direct audio input, where the person speaking holds or wears a microphone directly connected (via a wire) to your hearing aid. Many hearing aid wearers are reluctant to use a wired device. An alternative approach is to use instruments called assistive listening devices which transmit by FM (like a radio), infrared, or induction loop.

Realistic Expectations With New Hearing Aids

As I mentioned earlier, hearing aids are not new ears; they are electronic devices; they are not perfect; and for the most part, they do not eliminate background noise. Since many patients with sensorineural hearing loss deny the presence of a hearing impairment, or lack sufficient motivation, they often demand to be convinced of the improvement which hearing aids might offer. Since the main goal of amplification is to facilitate the ease of communication, don't be disappointed if you experience only minimal benefit during the initial trial with amplification.

The benefit derived from amplification may be subtle. That is, especially where only high frequency amplification occurs, there are only a few English language sounds in this range (such as /s/, /sh/, /t/, /th/, /f/, and /k/). Therefore, your hearing aids are designed to pick up only these consonants and since we're talking about relatively few sounds, the benefits of amplification may not be readily apparent. It's important to note here that even though we're speaking of a few sounds, these sounds are critically important. Remember that if you miss even one sound of one word, you could confuse the meaning of the message. On the other hand, the English language is, fortunately, quite redundant. If you do miss a sound or a word, try not to dwell on that word, because you may be able to pick up the meaning during the very next sentence. Remember that many sounds you miss are visible on the lips. Use your eyes! You don't have to be an accomplished lip-reader to obtain extremely valuable cues to supplement your listening. Mark Ross aptly discusses this later in Chapter 10.

You also need to recognize that prediction of guaranteed long-term benefit from amplification is difficult to determine. A period of initial adjustment and a learning process is required for most new hearing aid users. It may take several weeks before you adjust to the new pattern of sound and learn new "recognition" cues that you probably have not heard for a long time. As a new user, you need to be oriented to the world of amplification. You may require a gradual "break-in" wearing schedule (a few hours the first day, six hours the second, nine hours the third, etc.), or you may be encouraged to wear the hearing aid immediately during all your waking hours. You may require additional counseling and training, either individually, or in groups with other hearing impaired individuals and family members.

You must accept that time is required for adapting to hearing aids. Your ability to understand amplified speech can grow as much as three months following the use of a new hearing aid. Nearly all hearing health care professionals will give you a one month trial period with new hearing aids. If market conditions allow, trial periods may be extended. My advice is, if a trial period is not offered, take your business elsewhere!

It's important that you read the instruction manual that comes with your hearing aids. Hopefully, your provider will have told you everything you need to know about inserting and removing your hearing aids, checking the batteries, cleaning and maintaining the instruments, and using hearing aids with the telephone. But often, too much information can overload the brain! Take the hearing aids home, read the instruction manual, and then call your provider if you have any questions. Then go out and wear them in a variety of listening environments. When you return to your hearing health care provider, discuss the situations with which you may have had difficulty so that possible adjustments and fine-tuning can be achieved.

The Cost Of Hearing Aids

You may wonder why hearing aids cost what they do. They're sold in relatively low volume. That is, approximately 1.7 million hearing aids are sold annually for some 30 million hearing impaired people, as compared to several million stereos. Also, the amount of time and money spent by manufacturers on research and development is considerable. One manufacturer claims to have spent over 20 million dollars developing a single model.

Another factor considered in the cost of hearing aids is the amount of time spent by the provider with a patient is very significant. An average of five direct contact hours is spent during the first year a patient receives hearing aids. This time spent is critical for new users, particularly to facilitate adjustment.

Many hearing aids come with automatic loss and accidental damage insurance, depending on the manufacturer. If your hearing aids don't, talk with your hearing health care provider about insuring them. Also, the length of time your hearing aids remain under repair warranty can vary. Fortunately, most companies are fairly generous, and will include a repair warranty of one to two years in your initial cost. Some also offer extended warranties and loss and damage insurance. Ask your provider.

Conclusions

Now you have the facts, at least as they stand at the end of the 20th century. Remember, in order to have the best chance of succeeding with hearing aids, be patient with yourself and maintain realistic expectations. Even though dramatic technological improvements have been made, hearing aids do not restore normal hearing. Keep in mind that it's not necessary to hear every word said during conversations. You can supplement listening through your vision. And develop a trusting and open relationship with your hearing health care professional. Good luck and welcome to the world of better hearing!

CHAPTER EIGHT

Problem-Solving and Extending the Life of Your Hearing Aids

Thayne C. Smedley, Ph.D.

Ronald L. Schow, Ph.D.

Dr. Smedley is currently Professor of Audiology at Idaho State University in Pocatello. He received his Master of Science degree in Speech Pathology and Audiology from Utah State University, and a Ph.D. in Audiology from Stanford. He is nationally published in areas of hearing aid satisfaction and self-assessment issues. In his many years of clinical audiological practice, he has also dispensed hearing aids, and is currently invloved part-time in private practice. He has been Chief of the Audiology Section of the Veterans Administration Medical Center in San Francisco for nine years, and is Past-President of the Idaho Speech, Language and Hearing Association.

Dr. Schow, Professor of Audiology at Idaho State University, has specialized in audiological rehabilitation since earning his Doctorate from Northwestern University in 1974. He has twice been recognized at ISU with a campus-wide award as Outstanding Researcher. Dr. Schow has worked with many rehabilitation groups of hearing aid wearers, using satisfaction and other self-report questionnaires to measure successful outcomes. He's co-editor of a popular text on audiological rehabilitation now in its third edition. When he's not at ISU, he can often be found hiking and back-packing among the nearby Grand Tetons.

Hearing aids are electromechanical devices proven to be greatly beneficial to millions of people. Despite this fact, like any device, they are subject to breakdown. Consider that hearing aids typically are worn for long hours each day which places stress on electrical components and battery power. They exist in a relatively hostile environment of moisture, warm temperatures, especially with certain styles, and intrusive substances such as earwax, skin acids and oils. These substances may be healthy for the ear but potentially corrosive to hearing aids. For these reasons, no matter how well they're made, sooner or later they will stop working.

Hearing aid failure is almost always unpredictable and sometimes occurs at the most critical and inopportune time. Consider Fred's plight as he headed out the door for an early meeting with upper management on his job. Fred, who had worn hearing aids for several years, was a section supervisor in a large manufacturing firm.

Meetings with management occurred weekly but this one was especially important because it involved a review of company organization and possible restructuring of middle and upper management. The meeting would involve a lot of discussion which Fred needed to hear. He knew his supervisors were counting on his input. Fred was in line for a promotion and this could be a pivotal meeting for his career.

As he pulled his car out of the garage and headed down the street, he reached into his pocket for his hearing aid case, took out his hearing aids and slipped them comfortably into place. The car motor suddenly took on its normal drone as he turned the volume up. "Why is the right hearing aid sputtering?" he wondered. The aid had static and seemed a bit weak. Fred arrived at work and took his place in the conference room which was already filled with 20 of his co-workers. He was just a little late that morning so he took his place in the back of the room. But he knew he would be all right as long as he could hear. The hearing aid in his right ear continued to sputter and crackle. The company president opened the meeting and Fred's heart sank. His right hearing aid had gone dead. He hurried to throw in a fresh battery. The commotion interfered with the president's opening remarks and distracted his near-by associates; and to no avail. The hearing aid wouldn't respond. Frantically, Fred cranked up the left hearing aid to compensate. It promptly let out a wild squeal, attracting stares from his colleagues. He turned the left aid back down and sat there.

By this time, the president had finished his introductory remarks and had opened the meeting to discussion. What had the president said? Fred had caught only a small part of it and he fared no better with the other voices coming from different parts of the room. Because he was uncertain about what was being said, Fred did not feel part of the meeting. He was frustrated. He felt disappointed. He was angry. "I hate these hearing aids!" he mumbled to himself. It didn't help matters when his buddy George said to him on the way out, "Where were you today? I expected you to have a lot to say!"

Perhaps this episode strikes a resonate chord with you. Hearing aid failure can be upsetting, as Fred thought it was in his case. In less critical situations, a hearing aid that quits working may only produce frustration. At the very least, hearing aid breakdown is annoying.

This chapter addresses how to keep your hearing aids performing and how to spot the cause of malfunction early when breakdowns occur. We also include tips on preventive maintenance to improve hearing instrument reliability and longevity. Remember that some hearing aid failures will be unpreventable and beyond your control. Such failure will result in "down time" on your part and may require a send-off to the factory for repair. Also addressed will be sub-par performance from hearing aids which, although working, do not function as well as they might.

But first, a few words about hearing aid styles. Some styles of hearing aids are subject to more stress and abuse than others, and the approach you should take in troubleshooting hearing aid breakdowns can vary from one style to the next. Reasons for hearing aid failure which are related to a particular hearing aid style will be noted in each section. You need to be familiar with the basic hearing aid styles of which there are five. These styles are described in terms of their location on the ear or body, and for purposes of convenience are identified by acronyms. BB, BTE, ITE, ITC, and CIC (See Figure 7-1 in the previous chapter). In this chapter, minimal reference will be made to BB aids because so few of these are used today. Much of our instruction will be directed toward ITE and ITC aids because these represent the majority of styles in current use. Problems specific to CIC hearing aids will be highlighted because more and more hearing aids are being fit which are of this "deep canal" type.

As part of this introduction, a few words need to be said about hearing aid longevity. You may have asked, "How long will my hearing aids last?" Just as hearing aids will malfunction on occasion for reasons described above, it follows that they won't last indefinitely. This is true even for very expensive ones. For various reasons, cost being one of them, some users expect their instruments to last 10 to 15 years or more. Hearing aids that remain in useful service for this long are the exception rather than the rule. In fact, research has demonstrated that the typical hearing aid gets replaced about every five years. Also, some hearing aids are replaced not necessarily as a result of being worn out but due to changes in a person's hearing or because individuals may desire instruments of improved technology. In any case, you're well-advised to consider five years as the average life span of most hearing aids. All things considered, proper maintenance procedures will help to extend the longevity of any given hearing aid to its optimum potential.

Finally a comment about hearing aid reliability. In the following, we describe all the possible reasons hearing aids can fail. These should be read and studied carefully so you'll understand how hearing aids work and what to do if they quit. We present this outline of problem-solving techniques at the risk of giving you the impression that hearing aids are fragile, sensitive devices that will commonly fail and require unusual care and worry on your part. This is not at all the case. For the most part, today's hearing aids are exceptionally reliable and durable. They will serve your hearing needs day after day, year after year with rarely a breakdown.

Common Hearing Aid Problems and How to Solve Them

Kind of like your automobile, any number of problems can go wrong with a hearing aid, but for the most part, easy and relatively inexpensive remedies are available.

Dead and Defective Batteries

The inexperienced user is often disappointed by what is viewed as poor battery life. After all, watch batteries of approximately the same size last a year or more before replacement is necessary. Hearing aid battery life is related to two primary factors: the size (and storage capacity) of the battery and the amount of current draw required by the hearing aid. The larger the battery, the greater the storage capacity. However, the number of hours you will get from a battery depends on the current draw.

Hearing aid amplifiers simply draw heavy current loads, much heavier, for example, than those required for simple watch circuits, or even heart pacemakers for that matter. As a useful comparison, consider the common battery-operated flashlight. Interestingly, the typical flashlight uses a standard size D battery which has 1.5 volts, almost identical to the voltage of a hearing aid battery but of vastly larger size with greatly increased storage capacity. Even so, imagine how long a flashlight would work if it were used continuously for 16 hours a day as is required for hearing aids! The fact that hearing aid batteries maintain operation for long hours at a time, day after day, is quite impressive. Furthermore, battery efficiency has improved substantially in recent years. Today's batteries will keep a hearing aid going many days longer than the older style hearing aids (for example, BB-type) whose batteries were ten times larger! Signs of a failing battery are weak output, distortion, increased tendency of hearing aid feedback, intermittence and/or strange or unusual sounds such as static or fluttering (sometimes called "motorboating").

Weak and faulty batteries are a leading cause of hearing aid failure. In general, today's hearing aids require approximately 1.2 to 1.4 volts to operate properly. When a battery reaches 1.1 volts or less, the hearing aid will function poorly, if at all. The battery should then be replaced. In contrast to batteries of an earlier era, battery strength is sustained at a constant level until just a few hours before it dies, at which time it goes quickly. Older batteries used to lose power gradually over their life, requiring the user to adjust the volume at ever-increasingly higher levels to maintain proper output. This is not the case with today's batteries.

Anticipating the Dead Battery

So, in light of battery usage, how can you avoid hearing aid failure due to weak or dead batteries? First, you'll need to develop a replacement rhythm. Knowing the approximate time when a battery will go dead can decrease one of the sources of anxiety that may accompany hearing aid use. A replacement rhythm is most easily developed by marking a calendar each time a battery goes dead. A designation such as R-B or L-B for right aid or left aid batteries works nicely. If you use zinc-air batteries with a pull-tab, you can just as easily stick the tab on the corresponding date on the calendar and note it as right or left replacement. After a few weeks, you'll learn the replacement cycle required of the hearing aid and will become remarkably accurate in anticipating the impending demise of waning batteries. Calendar-marking may not be necessary after a few months, although for those with poor memory, it can be continued indefinitely.

For the technically oriented, an inexpensive battery tester can be purchased that will read the exact voltage strength of a new or used battery. This is probably a good investment because it allows you to determine if hearing aid failure is due to the battery itself.

Getting the most out of your batteries

Today's batteries have excellent shelf life, up to one year or more if kept in a cool, dry place. Refrigerating batteries, a common practice years ago, is unnecessary. Most batteries used today are of the zinc-air type which means a charge does not begin until a tab is removed from the face of the battery, allowing air to enter through tiny openings. Never remove the tab until the battery is to be inserted into the hearing aid.

To optimize battery longevity, disengage it when the aid is out of use for a period of time. The most common period of regular disuse for most wearers is overnight. When the aid is removed at bedtime, the easiest thing to do is simply open the battery compartment all the way and set the aid down on a dresser top or some other safe and convenient but accessible location. Avoid storing your hearing aids on a bed table or other similar location where children and/or dogs can get to them; otherwise they're easily lost or destroyed. It's not necessary to remove the battery from its compartment. Position the aid so that the door remains open and the battery remains in it. This will simplify hearing aid start-up the next morning. Just close the battery door and the aid is ready to go. If the aid is placed on the dresser carelessly, the battery may fall out. This isn't really a problem except that it creates an unnecessary inconvenience the next morning when the hearing aid battery must be located, oriented and reinserted. For individuals with limited vision or finger dexterity, this inconvenience can be significant. If you have an aid with the "toilet seat" door, you will have to remove the battery in order to preserve voltage.

Batteries in Backwards

The matter of inserting batteries, although not directly related to battery life, raises the question of another source of hearing aid failure. Batteries have a "negative" and "positive" polarity and therefore each side must be positioned correctly in the battery door to coincide with the electrical contact requirements of the circuit. The flashlight analogy cited earlier applies as well to battery orientation. We all know that a flashlight whose batteries are inserted incorrectly will not work. Manufacturers of hearing aids help with this problem as much as they can by marking a "+" sign on one side of the battery door to remind you that the positive side of the battery must be on that side. Because this "+" imprint is so small and for many impossible to see, the manufacturer also tailors the battery door to match the shape of the battery. A close look at any battery will disclose that batteries are perfectly flat on one side (the positive side) and beveled on the other (the negative side). The battery door is similarly configured and should be studied by new users in its open position, under a magnifying lamp if necessary, to learn these identifying characteristics. Then you can position the battery appropriately in your fingers and insert it correctly with confidence.

Please note that with the battery in place, if the door doesn't close readily with only a minimum of force, this is often a sign the battery is in backwards. When this happens, reverse the battery and try again. In any case, *do not force the battery into place*. Doing so can damage the hearing aid. At this writing, some manufacturers are producing hearing aid circuits that will accept batteries placed in either position. This modification is in response to the difficulties some users have with battery insertion. This technological improvement may be the standard someday with all hearing aids.

Finally, never insert the battery into its place by accidentally sliding it beneath the battery door. By-passing the battery door will usually not damage the hearing aid but may likely jam the battery in place and require a trip to your provider to have it removed.

Battery Disposal

Naturally, every user likes to get the most hours possible from every battery. To do this, some people will remove batteries that show the earliest signs of weakening and save them for later use after they've recovered some of their charge. It's true that near-spent batteries will self-rejuvenate to a degree after removal from a hearing aid and may provide power for an extra day or so. This strategy of holding onto spent batteries, however, has several problems. First, it can give you a false sense of security. Hearing aid batteries with weak voltages can fail at any moment. Secondly, and of greater concern, these batteries sometimes get mixed in with the fresh batteries. The result is confusion and frustration if a bad battery is picked up and inserted in the hearing aid when it's thought to be good.

Finally, re-using worn batteries is a poor practice because the savings associated with this practice are not really worth the bother. Consider the following: assume a battery lasts two weeks and costs $1.00. If a user gets two extra days per battery by recycling spent batteries, the result would be four extra days use per month. The daily cost of batteries using two per month at a cost of $1.00 per battery is about 6 cents ($2.00 divided by 31 days). So, four extra days at 6 cents/day is 24 cents savings per month, or less than $3.00 per year. A savings of $3.00 per year is clearly not worth the hassle of keeping track of used batteries. This also holds for binaural users who might save approximately $6.00 per year. Our advice is, when zinc-air batteries go dead, throw them away. (Silver-oxide batteries, although not commonly used today, can be recycled.) Also, never leave bad batteries lying around where children can get them. Batteries can do serious damage if ingested.*

Conserving Battery Life

Some hearing aid users concerned with operating costs will turn their hearing aids off when they "don't need to hear." Such individuals feel they get increased longevity with this strategy, analogous to the "turn off the lights when not in use" philosophy. While there may be some justification for this practice in special circumstances (for example, while working in a noisy shop for a few hours), a habit of turning hearing aids on and off "as needed" is not recommended. You can never tell when an important auditory event will come along, such as another person's voice or a warning signal. You don't want to be inconsiderate of others by shutting off your "antenna" so you hear them only when you want to. Furthermore, it's important to be aware of the rich assortment of environmental sounds that keep us in touch with the world.

Stockpiling Fresh Batteries

With today's batteries, is there anything wrong with storing a reasonable supply? If you see a two-for-one battery special, it's tempting to take advantage of this offer and save money but we give you this caution: such "sale batteries" are sometimes promoted to get rid of old stock and might more correctly be termed "stale batteries."

If you're inclined to store a supply of batteries, our advice is to investigate the manufacture date and then purchase no more than six months' supply at a time. Beyond this period, full storage life of the batteries might be compromised. Also, you just might decide to change hearing aids before the supply is used up, resulting in an over-supply of batteries that may no longer be of the appropriate size. People who travel are well-advised to purchase an adequate supply of batteries before taking a trip, especially if traveling overseas. Try to avoid situations where you must make a purchase of unfamiliar brands which may be of poor quality or irregular size.

The Defective Battery

Present-day batteries are very reliable as a rule and you can usually depend on a fresh battery working as it should. Occasionally, however, a new battery or a whole pack will be defective. Your

*Should this occur, call the National Button Battery Ingestion Hotline, telephone number (202) 625-3333 for assistance.

provider will gladly exchange them for a fresh package.

Earwax Obstruction

Another leading cause of hearing aid failure is wax blockage. The technical name for common earwax is cerumen. It's produced by glands (actually called ceruminous glands) in the outer ear roughly one-third of the way down the ear canal. The product of these glands is a pasty substance, usually light brown or tan in color and bitter in taste. (Take our word on this one!) Cerumen is believed to exist in the ear canal to discourage flies and insects from entering this opening.

The degree of wax generated in the canal varies greatly from one person to the next. On average, men experience more wax build-up than women. Some women, however, can produce large amounts of cerumen, as can children. For reasons not clearly understood, some individuals generate little or no wax. If you're presently unaware of the wax condition in your ears, your physician or hearing health care provider can readily inform you of this after examination with an otoscope (ear light).

Hearing aid users must continually be on the lookout for adverse effects of earwax. When hearing aids are inserted into the ear canals, (or earmolds in the case of BTE hearing aids), they can slide alongside or directly into accumulated wax. The fresher the wax, the softer and more easily it can get pushed into the sound bore (receiver) of an aid. A thin smear of earwax over the receiver tube will shut the aid down instantly.

Preventing Wax Build-up

The first defense against wax build-up is regular cleaning of your ear canals by a physician or audiologist, or as simple as it sounds, in a shower by direct spray into the canals. The cautions here are to be careful of the water pressure, and be certain you don't have a hole in the eardrum, or any other condition which might prevent such easy management of earwax.

Hearing instrument specialists are not usually trained to remove earwax, and some audiologists may not offer this service—although current thinking is that wax removal is within the scope of practice for audiologists. In any case, you are well-advised to locate a person or office that will provide this service as needed. Attempting to control build-up of earwax by regular use of cotton swabs is not recommended. Aside from the possibility of doing physical damage to the ear canal or drum (the "don't put anything in your ear smaller than your elbow" concept), cotton swabs will usually only serve to pack the wax deeper with each attempt. By looking into the ear, professionals can readily discern the cotton swab users, as the wax shows a nicely formed concave surface down in the ear canal.

Some hearing aid users with chronic wax problems may find regular use of "ear lavage" effective. Equipment along with instructions for home use are available in many hearing care offices and drug stores. Wax softeners for use prior to cleaning can also be purchased. Some people may be uncomfortable squirting water into the ear canal. A discussion with your physician would be advisable before attempting it. The main problem with this type of treatment is the difficulty knowing when the wax is all out.

The second defense against wax blockage is utilization of some type of wax guard. There are a number of commercially available products which suit this purpose, the most common of which is a tiny wire coil inserted into the receiver tube (See Figure 8-1). Many manufacturers now provide such a device as original equipment. Directly, or under magnification if necessary, you can look into the sound opening of the hearing aid and spot this coil if it's there. Two other devices include an adhesive patch over the receiver opening; or a "trap-door" style guard. All such devices should be discussed thoroughly with your hearing health care provider who can properly service them.

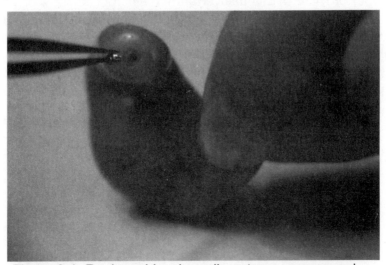

Figure 8-1: Replaceable wire coil captures earwax and prevents it from entering receiver of hearing aid.(Removal with tweezers recommended only by your provider.)

Responsibility for Wax Maintenance

This is not to say that whoever dispensed your hearing aids has primary responsibility to keep them free of earwax. You need to develop a daily habit of inspecting the end of the hearing aid where the sound comes out and looking for wax blockage. If accumulation is noticed, this wax can be readily removed in most cases.

When and How to Remove Wax

The best time to inspect hearing aids for wax is at the close of the day. At this time, any accumulated wax will still be soft and more easily removed. If you use the Band-Aid style guard, you can wipe across it gently. After a few days if you observe the cushion separating from the adhesive backing, remove it altogether and replace. If used properly, you'll never need to clean out the receiver (loud speaker) which is the rubber housing hole at the tip of an aid. If your hearing aids don't have the wire coil in them, you may use a device known as a wax loop (See Figure 8-2). This is merely a wire looped around the end of a piece of plastic. Gently insert it into the receiver tube, turn it one full rotation, then remove. Avoid picking or poking. If your hearing aid has the wax coil, be careful not to push it too far into the tubing, which could short-circuit the aid. Clean any debris from the loop. Nightly cleaning has the added advantage of keeping the receiver tube open for more adequate ventilation and drying. Review this procedure carefully and thoroughly with your provider so that inadvertently you don't damage your hearing aids by cramming the wax loop into the wrong opening (such as the microphone port on the face of the hearing aid) or too deeply into the receiver port which can damage the speaker diaphragm. Additionally, a wax tool that is a little too large to fit readily into the receiver tube can push the tube itself down into the shell of the hearing aid. This will

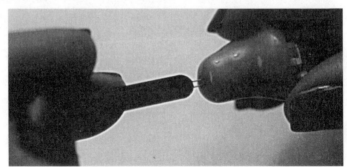

Figure 8-2: Use of a probe wire for cleaning the receiver tubing of a shell-type hearing aid.

damage the instrument, often causing it to squeal, resulting in needed repairs.

Wax should also be removed from hearing aid vents. Because vents are longer, often running the length of the earpiece or earmold, they're not as easily cleaned. Only recently have manufacturers supplied an appropriate cleaning tool suitable for vents, and then only for CIC aids. Figure 8-3 shows the tool. It's rather flimsy, necessarily of small gauge, and quite fragile. It does the job, however. You can also use a stiff piece of heavy duty fish line of the appropriate gauge. Some people have resorted to the use of wires of various gauges to ream out vents. Wire should be used with caution as it can crack the shell. Large vents are less likely to get plugged up and much easier to clean. Pipe cleaners work extremely well for large vents, such as those commonly found in ITEs. Your provider will have suggestions for obtaining these and other suitable tools for cleaning.

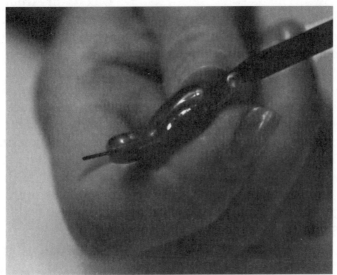

Figure 8-3: Demonstration of cleaning a CIC vent with a probe wire.

Sometimes, wax build-up becomes dry and flaky before it's removed. When this happens, a good brushing of the hearing aid openings can be helpful in addition to use of the wire loop. When brushing, always hold the hearing aid upside down so that wax particles fall out of, rather than down into, the hearing aid (See Figure 8-4). Also, keep your brush clean so that wax particles which collect in the bristles from previous brushing aren't injected inadvertently into the openings.

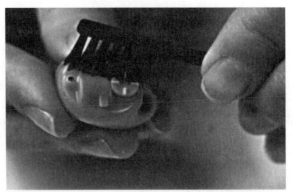
Figure 8-4: Demonstration of the proper
use of brushing (viewed from beneath).

Moisture

Handling moisture problems will depend on what type of hearing aids you own. The use of water to remove wax or dirt from any part of the hearing aid itself is generally inadvisable. Moisture is a natural enemy to electronic devices. The use of a dry cloth or tissue to wipe clean the outside surface of the hearing aid is the only recommended cleaning practice.

With regard to BTE style hearing aids, earmolds used with these instruments must be removed from the hearing aids before cleaning. They can be soaked in a solution of soap and warm water, gently scrubbed clean, then completely dried before re-connecting to the hearing aid. The only method we recommend for drying is the hand-held, forced-air blower which simply pumps air through the tubing. Failure to do this will risk moisture seepage into the aid.

Ear Discomfort

Like pressure on the feet from a tight fitting pair of new shoes, hearing aids can occasionally be uncomfortable. Unlike feet, however, such discomfort in the ear is not tolerated well. Hearing aid-related ear pain can distract from intended amplification. The comment, "I think I'm hearing better with hearing aids, but I can't tell for sure because of the discomfort," illustrates the problem. Discomfort associated with hearing aid use usually has a specific anatomical site of origin but a widespread reaction. That is, a tight-fitting earmold may cause specific tenderness in one spot in the ear canal but in time the sensation can radiate.

Causes of Ear Discomfort

The most common cause of ear discomfort is an ill-fitting earmold (in the case of BTE) or hearing aid shell (in the case of ITE, ITC or CIC). Earpieces are fabricated from impressions taken of your ear. Usually they'll fit precisely. They're designed to fit snugly but not uncomfortably. It should be realized, however, that your degree of hearing loss will have a bearing on the tightness. Severe hearing losses must have a tight fit to prevent feedback (whistling).

There are two causes for ear discomfort which can result from a poorly fitting hearing aid or earmold. Either the earpiece was made improperly, or is incorrectly positioned in the ear. Impressions can and usually do provide exact replicas of the ear canal. This is because most providers are experienced in taking ear impressions. Occasionally, however, impressions can be distorted during preparation, while in transit to the laboratory, or during fabrication.

Another factor affecting comfort has to do with jaw movement. In some cases ear pain is caused or aggravated by movement of the jaw when earpieces are in place. For many, movement of the jaw can have significant influence on the shape of the canal. This is really quite normal. The effects of jaw movement can be felt by placing the "pinkie" finger deep in the ear canal while moving the jaw. (Try it while you're reading this). This movement arises from the joint of the lower jaw called, technically, the temporomandibular joint, or simply TMJ. Even though earmolds may have reflected accurate impressions of the canal, the resulting earpieces may not "give" when the jaw and ear canal are moving, as when talking or chewing. If you suspect a poorly fitting earmold or hearing aid due to influences of the TMJ, you may want to discuss this matter with your hearing care professional.

The second most common cause of ear discomfort is the earpiece which is placed incorrectly in the ear. Figure 8-5 shows both correct and incorrect insertion. Earmolds which have been accurately fabricated can cause ear pain if not inserted correctly. When placing the earmold or hearing aid in the ear, you must make certain the device is "seated" into its exact location or else it'll create pressure points in the canal. Difficulties with correct placement can be a fairly common problem, especially for new users. Those who use BTE hearing aids, for example, must make sure the entire earmold is properly placed. A common problem here is when the earmold is inserted into the canal, the uppermost portion isn't tucked into the groove of skin at the top of the ear. This incomplete placement can shift the angle of the earmold just enough to create a tender spot down in the canal. ITE users can have the same problem.

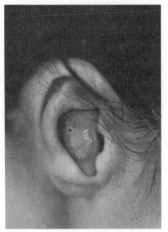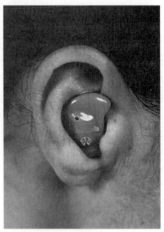

Figure 8-5: The correct (left) and incorrect (right) placement of a shell-type hearing aid.

Those who try CIC instruments may experience some fitting and placement problems initially. The deeper a hearing aid is placed in the canal, the more sensitive the canal tissue. Some users are simply reluctant to push an aid fully into the canal, fearful that doing so will cause pain. This is understandable. Also, there can be concern the aid can be pushed too deeply into the canal and cause damage. This also is a logical concern. However, ear canals tend to be carrot-shaped (that is, the deeper into the canal, the narrower the opening) and the aid cannot be pushed without discomfort beyond its appropriate location. With practice, however, you will soon get a "feel" for the exact location of the aid and should be able to insert it correctly with confidence and without discomfort. If placement difficulties aren't easily resolved, practicing proper insertion of the hearing aid in the presence and under the watchful eye of your provider is helpful and reassuring.

Correcting a Fitting Problem

Ear discomfort associated with a new set of hearing aids can be either transitory or persistent. If you're a new user, you should understand that initial discomfort of a slight degree can be expected. Normally, we wear nothing inside the ear canal, so tolerating that first earpiece will require some adjustment. Such discomfort will subside substantially or be completely gone after only a few days. The new shoe example cited earlier will apply here as well.

Discomfort which persists after going through an initial adjustment period is another matter. Unrelenting discomfort present each time the hearing aid is worn should certainly be noted in follow-up visits with your clinical audiologist or hearing instrument specialist. During such visits your provider will either need to modify the earpiece by grinding or buffing, or remake the fitting by taking a new impression. It's helpful here to note that in most situations of poor fit, satisfactory corrections can be made right in the office. Also, please be aware that most users don't experience these initial difficulties at all and "hit the ground running" with new hearing aids. Often, we hear in the office, "I forget they're even in my ears!"

Plugged Up Vents

A vent in an earmold or hearing aid is simply an open passageway or tube that extends from the front of the earpiece to the tip. It almost always exits the tip very close to the sound opening (receiver tube). Except in the case of more significant hearing loss, a vent will always be present. The diameter of the vent may be either large or small. In general, hearing aids fit to people with mild loss will have large vents while those fit to individuals with more severe losses will have smaller vents. They're usually placed in earmolds or hearing aid shells by manufacturers. They can also be placed there or modified by your provider. Vents should always be kept open to perform their intended function.

Purposes of Vents

Vents are placed in earpieces for four rather important reasons. They allow sounds that you may hear normally to enter the ear canal directly without being amplified. You don't want to block the ear to sounds which you hear normally. Vents that serve this purpose are usually fairly large and obvious. This type of vent is very helpful if your hearing loss affects only higher pitches (technically called frequencies).

The second purpose of venting is to reduce amplification of unwanted sounds. Often these are low-pitched tones which you may already hear normally. Experienced, and sometimes even new users will report hearing better when their provider enlarges the vent by drilling. This diminishes low-pitch bothersome background sounds. Hearing aids and earmolds fit to those with more severe loss will require smaller vents.

A third purpose of venting, perhaps the most important in some fittings, is to decrease the acoustic effects of your own voice. You'll readily identify this as the objectionable sounds of your own voice while the ears are blocked off. This is called the "occlusion effect," as described in the previous chapter. It's the "my voice sounds like I'm talking in a barrel" effect.

Moisture Problems

As noted earlier, ear canals can produce a degree of moisture which can affect hearing aid performance. Like the problem of earwax, the amount of moisture present in human ear canals can vary widely from person to person. Your activity level and climatic conditions in which hearing aids are worn are two of the more common variables affecting moisture build-up. People with high levels of physical activity who perspire easily can be more prone to moisture problems than those who lead a more sedentary life. Moreover, a moisture problem can be further aggravated by conditions of high humidity. Moisture build-up can result from either internal or external sources. Internal sources are those related to the condition of the auditory canal while the latter refers to liquids which arise from outside the ear, as those, for example, associated with rain or severe perspiration.

The Effects of Moisture

While BTE-type hearing aids, if maintained properly, can outlast in-the-shell types, they tend to have the worst problem with moisture. Water vapors arising from the canal condense in the connecting tube. When these vapors reach a region outside the canal of slightly cooler temperature, condensation converts to small droplets of water which appear as tiny bubbles in the tube. The accumulation of enough water droplets can be sufficient to close the tube and shutdown amplification.

Externally-produced moisture surprisingly is less of a problem. Rain water, unless very severe or persistent, usually runs around the ear and off the head with little or no adverse affects. A worse condition, especially for BTE use, exists for the person who perspires a lot. With such individuals, beads of perspiration form in the hair along the top of the hearing aid. In time, this moisture can seep into the cracks and openings along the upper surface of the hearing aid and eventually affect operation. The case of the postal worker comes to mind whose daily walking route involved extreme outside weather conditions. The operation of his BTE hearing aid was little affected by rain water which was easily diverted by wearing a wide-brimmed hat. Heavy perspiration, however, caused predictable shutdowns during workdays of extreme heat and high humidity. It's worth noting here that proper care and maintenance will reduce mechanical problems associated with moisture.

Hearing aids of the type worn in the ear have less difficulty with moisture build-up. Externally produced moisture with in-the-shell-type hearing aids tends to flow around rather than into the ear as a rule. Also, the further the aid is placed inside the canal, the less the problem as moisture from the canal lining has less of an opportunity to get into the receiver tube. Therefore, CIC's are the least affected by internal and external moisture.

Resolving Moisture Problems

The point was emphasized earlier that moisture and electronic devices are a poor mix. To every extent possible, moisture in the region of the ear must be avoided. This means, to state the obvious, that hearing aids are not to be worn while showering, bathing, or swimming. They should also be removed before getting into a hot-tub, steam room, or while participating in water sports of any kind. These precautions apply equally well to moisture-related exposures such as spray paint, spray deodorant, hair sprays, and most aerosols. Chemicals in these particles are particularly destructive because they leave permanent residues which build up over time. With repeated use, they are certain to cause eventual hearing aid failure and permanent damage.

When hearing aids are unavoidably exposed to moisture, as with individuals who must work outdoors, extra precautions must be used. In the case of the postal worker cited earlier, a simple plastic sleeve slipped over each BTE instrument resolved the problem without significantly affecting performance. Some hearing aids are constructed specifically with watertight gaskets and are more weatherproof than others. Actually, most recent vintage hearing aids are surprisingly resistant to water damage and function in a variety of situations without intermittence, especially if they can thoroughly dry out overnight. In this regard, hearing aids should be left in the open air when stored overnight, especially if moisture build-up is a problem. The use of dry-packs which absorb moisture can also be used to advantage during storage. These dry-packs are inexpensive and available from your hearing care professional.

Other drying techniques may also be tried. One recent BTE user who had a chronic problem with moisture solved it by dangling his hearing aids (overnight) *upside down* by the earmolds from a homemade wire hanger. In this position, moisture was more readily able to escape from the hearing aids than when they were stored lying flat which tended to trap the moisture.

Finally, it should be noted that hearing aid failure due to moisture is not always easy to diagnose. Except for water vapor forming in the tube of BTE hearing aids which is readily visible, moisture is difficult to observe. If hearing aid stoppage is found to be unrelated to the more obvious causes, such as faulty batteries or wax blockage, then moisture build-up should be suspected. The use of drying procedures previously described should help isolate this problem. Also, perhaps with the help of your provider, you could check your daily routine. For example, it will do little good to faithfully dry out hearing aids overnight if every morning after they're inserted you apply a healthy portion of hair spray!

Poor Battery Life

Shortened battery life will result most likely from one of three possibilities: the battery is defective and has a weakened charge; the hearing aid is defective and draws current in excess of what it should; or the battery routinely is left in operation in the hearing aid during periods of disuse (for example, overnight). Users who are always careful to disconnect the battery overnight can usually assume a defective aid in the situation of poor battery life. While batteries can be faulty on occasion, as noted earlier, most commonly it will be the hearing aid itself at fault. When this happens, the likely solution is factory repair.

Before an aid is returned to your provider with this problem, it's wise to verify that your present batteries in use are in fact good. Because battery life can vary somewhat within acceptable limits, we recommend taking action with the hearing aid only when battery life is consistently one-half of what it regularly has been or should be. This would help to confirm a defective hearing aid. Otherwise, you might be dealing simply with variability in longevity among batteries.

The Problem of Intermittence

We have touched upon a variety of hearing aid problems to this point, each of which can cause some degree of intermittence: a bad battery, a fleck of earwax, a little moisture. In addition, hearing aids can develop intermittence from other causes though these may be less frequent.

Dirty Volume Control

Hearing aids that still use volume controls (some current hearing aids don't) operate on the basis of metal contact points that slide against each other in normal operation. You can almost feel movement in the contacts as you rotate the volume wheel up and down. These contact points can become corroded with dirt or other residue that will not allow current to pass. This may occur when the volume control is in certain positions where corrosion is the worst. The result is an aid that goes on and off or even produces a very audible static noise as it's being adjusted. If you experience this problem, we recommend you rotate the volume control knob in continuous movements back and forth between low and high power up to 20-30 times. If this does not resolve the problem, it will require factory cleaning and/or repair.

Dirty Battery Contacts

Battery contact points can also become corroded and create similar problems. As with the volume control, dust, moisture, and earwax are the primary culprits. Corroded contacts in the battery compartment result in intermittent or stopped current flow which has a direct effect on hearing aid output. Corroded battery contacts are also quite difficult for you to clean and will require office or factory servicing.

The Problem of Oily Skin

Some individuals with oily skin have battery contact problems. During routine handling and insertion of batteries, oily residue can be transferred from finger tips to the surfaces of the battery and adversely affect contact pickup. Such oily film can cause intermittence. If you suspect this problem, replace batteries while holding them with an ordinary tissue to prevent their surface "contamination," or be careful to wash your hands thoroughly before handling them.

Summary

It should be noted in summary that during regular use, it's

impossible to prevent a certain amount of contamination of hearing aids from elements in the environment. Sooner or later these elements are bound to affect instrument performance. The auto mechanic, for example, who works in a greasy, dust-laden environment is highly susceptible to hearing aid corrosion. Intermittence and frequent servicing should be expected when hearing aids are used in such unfavorable environments.

Poor Telephone Reception

If hearing and understanding speech are difficult face to face, even with hearing aids, then telephone reception will be similarly difficult. Likewise, if your hearing aids allow you to function well in a face to face situation, you should converse with little difficulty on the telephone.

At the outset, it should be noted that some people have no difficulty hearing on the telephone without their hearing aid. This is because the telephone system has some built-in amplification, and a telephone held closely to the ear can provide adequate pickup while blocking out some background interference. Individuals with greater loss will need additional amplification to hear well on the telephone. On the other hand, those with severe to profound loss may be unable to converse at all on the telephone, with or without amplification. To explore what telephone amplifying devices are available to you, see Chapter 13.

Whether you use hearing aids or not for the telephone, if you're in the presence of noise, cover the mouthpiece each time after you speak. This prevents undesirable room noise from traveling into your telephone receiver and being amplified into your own ear (or hearing aid), adding confusion to what you may already be finding difficult to hear.

The Telecoil Circuit

One mechanism developed to improve telephone reception that has been available for many years is the telecoil (short for telephone coil). Not all hearing aids have them. If yours has it, you'll see some designation or switch on the case. BTE-type hearing aids with this device will have a switch position labeled "T." In-the-shell hearing aids may simply have a manual two-way switch. Because the telecoil circuit requires extra space, smaller hearing instruments such as the ITC or especially CIC will not have them.

Telecoil circuits work by processing electromagnetic waves

produced by the telephone receiver (a process known in electronics as induction). When the hearing aid switch is on "T," a special wire coil is activated within the hearing aid circuit in place of the microphone. The only sounds that will come through the hearing aid in this position are what you hear through the telephone. Background noise near the telephone, for example, is unamplified which is a big advantage. Hearing aids with T-coils (as they're called) should work on nearly all currently available telephones. Telecoils can be quite satisfactory for mild to moderate hearing losses.

Successful Use of the Telecoil Circuit

Review of your Operator's Manual will familiarize you with the telephone setting. If the hand-switch on the aid is not set to the telephone mode, only the regular microphone will pick up sound which may provide inadequate reception. To get the best reception from the telecoil, the receiver of the telephone must be positioned within the most sensitive area of the hearing aid. To find this position, simply move the telephone earpiece around the ear during conversation until the voice comes in loudest. Your provider will be more than happy to demonstrate this procedure on an office telephone.

Other Tips for Improved Telephone Listening

Selection of the most appropriate hearing device is the first step toward successful telephone use. The clinical audiologist or hearing instrument specialist should be consulted during the selection process so that your individual needs are given full consideration. For some, telephone use is of little consequence. To others, it may be critical. For this latter group all possible telephone options need to be carefully explored.

The next most important step is practice. Optimum telephone pickup is often achieved only after periods of trial and error. When asked about telephone use, an occasional hearing aid user will say, "I tried it once but it didn't work." You'll need more patience than that. Don't expect to get your best results after only one or two attempts. Practice is especially important here and the best way to get practice is to prearrange a long telephone conversation with a friend or relative. Explain that you're experimenting over the telephone with your new hearing aids. A patient listener will allow you to try your hearing aid in a variety of telephone positions (or perhaps hearing aid settings as well) until you achieve optimum reception. Such practice will result in success with the telephone in a wide majority of cases. Also realize that poor telephone reception can be the fault of the telephone in isolated cases.

Hearing Aid Squeal (Acoustic Feedback)

Feedback is the term we use for the high-pitched squeal commonly associated with amplifiers which have microphones and loudspeakers connected to them. This is the case with hearing aids (See Chapter 7). The squeal is caused by amplified sound that radiates from the speaker, is inadvertently picked up by the microphone and gets continuously re-amplified. The same thing can happen in an auditorium when the loudspeaker and microphone are too close together, or the amplifier volume is set too high. The hearing aid is said to "go into oscillation," and the squealing sound coming from the loudspeaker is the result. Feedback can be avoided when the sound coming out the loudspeaker is prevented from reaching the microphone.

In the case of hearing aids, the pathway of sound from the loudspeaker opening (receiver) to the microphone input is along the side of the hearing aid or earmold in the ear canal, or through a vent. If the earmold or shell-type hearing aid fit snugly into the ear, and the vent is not too large, sound is unable to leak out and reach the microphone located outside the ear canal, in which case the aid won't squeal. When hearing aids or earmolds fit too loosely in the canal, the opposite can result. In general, a loose-fitting hearing aid or earmold is more likely to squeal than a tight one. Also, a high-powered hearing aid will have a greater tendency to feedback than a low-powered aid and therefore will require a tighter fitting earmold. Competent hearing care professionals realize that the size and placement of hearing aid vents must be determined with the utmost regard to the potential for feedback.

Acceptable Versus Unacceptable Feedback

We want to emphasize that acoustic feedback is a natural phenomenon of amplifiers and not of concern, in and of itself. Feedback is to be expected, for example, when a hearing aid is "on" and held in a cupped hand. It does no damage to use feedback in this way to tell if the hearing aid is working. Similarly, it's usually not a problem to purposely cup the hand to the ear and listen for the "beep" as the hand is moved toward and away from the ear. Many users test the hearing aid in this way to be sure it's on. Others will rotate the volume control to the position of feedback during adjustment. Here again, this is no problem. These are all examples of predictable and acceptable feedback.

Unacceptable feedback is the type that spontaneously rings without warning or provocation, that happens, for example, while you're chewing, brushing your hair, scratching the side of your head, or tilting your head downward. This latter movement causes a slight shift in the position of the hearing aid, sometimes just enough to allow sound to leak out. The squeal associated with all of these activities can be vexing. Feedback of the unacceptable kind also occurs when you try to turn the volume of the hearing aid up to a more desirable level but cannot because the aid starts to squeal. At this volume position, with you attempting to extract the last decibel of sound possible, the aid is on the verge of feedback and will squeal at the least little disturbance. These are examples of feedback which you will not want to tolerate. Almost all of them can be corrected.

Earwax and Feedback

Feedback can occur anytime sound is deflected toward the microphone. Normal eardrums tend to absorb energy so that if an earpiece is reasonably snug, leakage is minimal and feedback doesn't occur. Earwax, on the other hand, seems to absorb very little sound and will bounce the sound right back out of the canal toward the microphone. Therefore, individuals who experience unexplained feedback should have their ears checked for wax build-up.

Solving the Feedback Problem

People with the most severe hearing loss provide the greatest challenge to their provider when it comes to feedback control. Most of it is still manageable. As noted earlier, a first consideration in dealing with feedback is to ensure that your ear canals are clear of wax. This does not usually require a medical evaluation each time the ears need to be checked. The audiologist or hearing instrument specialist can do the job just as well and usually at no cost. If the canals are obstructed, your provider may charge a fee to remove wax, or if necessary refer you to a physician. You may want to insist that examination of your ear canals be a part of regular office hearing aid check-ups.

Given clear canals, the next obvious concern in dealing with feedback is the fit of the hearing aids. The most common cause of all feedback problems is poorly fitting earpieces. Sometimes the hearing aid or earmold are ill-fitting from the very beginning. Hearing aids that have been used for several years without a feedback problem can gradually develop it as the aid "loosens up" in the ear. This results from two possibilities. If you wear BTE's with earmolds, the earmolds can shrink and change shape. Also, tissues along the wall of the canal can gradually give way to small but persistent pressure associated with the instrument. (The shoe and foot analogy again.) This problem of increasing tendency for feedback is pronounced in children whose bodies undergo relatively rapid changes. Therefore, more frequent remakes can be expected with this age group to control feedback, especially in cases of severe loss.

Feedback with New Purchases

If you have purchased new hearing aids that squeal or act like they're always on the verge of squealing, or do when volume is moved up to a desired level, insist on getting the problem corrected—the sooner the better. Correcting a feedback problem with a new fitting is most easily done during the initial issuance.

Some feedback problems can be corrected readily in the office while the more severe cases may require a remake of the fitting. This will involve, of course, taking new impressions and going without the hearing aid for a brief time. But the temporary inconvenience will be well worth it. Whatever you do, don't allow the problem to go uncorrected, thinking, "Well, in time it'll probably straighten itself out." A feedback problem will rarely go away on its own. If anything, it usually gets worse. Left unattended, a feedback problem can result in a fitting that is highly unsatisfactory.

Feedback and Telephone Use

Feedback occurs most often when some object is placed next to the hearing aid. This object can be a telephone, your own hand or even a nearby wall or other flat surface. Feedback is not a problem with hearing aids (having a telecoil circuit) when the switch is in the "T" position. However, it is a common problem with standard hearing aids. Careful positioning of the telephone which usually involves removing the receiver a slight distance from the ear or tilting it on a slight angle will eliminate the feedback and still allow adequate reception. Some hearing aids are less susceptible to feedback than others. CIC-type instruments, for example, are the most feedback-free of any. A commercial product that is a thin, donut-shaped, sponge-like device can be purchased from your provider and attached to the receiver of the telephone to reduce feedback.

Static and Other Unwanted Sounds

Be assured that unless you happen to be listening to an old radio badly tuned to the station, internally generated static of any kind is

154

abnormal and in need of correction. Static resulting from internal causes means that the noise is created from some problem inside the hearing aid or telephone and not existing in the environment.

Recall that for the hearing aid to have clear sound, adequate battery voltage must be maintained. Likewise, current drawn from the battery must be appropriate or the hearing aid can produce strange sounds. In cases of low voltage or dirty contacts, cleaning or replacing the battery, or servicing the contact points in the battery door should correct the problem. Moisture and dirt in the volume control or other switches can also cause static. Here again, cleaning and regular servicing will help.

Sometimes strange sounds including static-type noise come through the hearing aid even though it's relatively clean and the batteries are fresh. This can be caused by defective components in the amplifier. These components can wear out in time and require replacement. Also, some hearing aids will pick up strange sounds that radiate from electrical appliances or light fixtures, especially fluorescent. Such sounds are externally generated. Hearing aids that pick up these kinds of unwanted sounds seem to be less of a problem now than with older hearing aids.

Another source of unexplained sound coming through a hearing aid that should be mentioned here are those sounds in the environment which you may have forgotten existed or you've not heard for a long time. New users often pick up on these *new noises* right away. One such person complained, "Since I bought these hearing aids, I hear a terrible noise in my kitchen I never heard before. It's mostly constant but sometimes it goes off for awhile. What's wrong with these hearing aids?" A courtesy home visit revealed that what she was hearing was the compressor of her old refrigerator! Obviously, she hadn't heard this noise for a long time. Other sounds to which you'll need to become re-acclimated are common noises associated with motion, like paper rattling, water running, utensils dropping on a plate, and wind.

Wind Noise

If you spend a lot of time outdoors, wind noise can be especially bothersome. If so, you might want to investigate a CIC-style fitting which will eliminate or greatly reduce wind sounds. For non-CIC instruments, a "windhood" or "windscreen" can be installed that can also help the problem. Discuss these options with your provider.

Background Noise

The single largest complaint of hearing aid users is difficulty hearing in the presence of background noise. Unfortunately, hearing aids, even the most expensive ones, have difficulty separating the sounds and voices you want to hear from those in which you have no interest. So you'll have to learn to put up with a certain amount of noise just as people with normal hearing do. The new programmable hearing aids do offer some relief for those who must function regularly in noisy situations.

Preventive Hearing Aid Maintenance

Few consumer purchases have any faster rate of depreciation and limited resale value than hearing aids. Stated differently, from an economic standpoint your hearing aids are of no value to anyone but you. For this reason and because they're expensive to replace, it makes good sense to service them on a regular basis. Systematic maintenance will reduce repair costs, lessen the number of "down" times, and most importantly extend the life of your hearing instruments. What follows is a brief list of maintenance procedures that will help you to accomplish this:

- **Clean Your Hearing Aids Daily:** This is best accomplished by first wiping the hearing aids with a dry cloth or tissue to remove wax, oil and moisture from the surface. Then lightly dry-brush all components using the wax removal techniques described earlier, and remove wax from the receiver and vent tubes. This cleaning should be done daily, preferably at bedtime.
- **Proper Storage:** Place hearing aids in a safe, convenient and protected location, being certain to disengage the battery door in a manner recommended previously. Sticking hearing aids in pockets or at the bottom of purses without a protective container exposes them to dirt and dust that can eventually do damage. Dust-free carrying cases are provided with nearly all new hearing aids. You should have this case available when necessary. If moisture build-up is a concern, store the hearing aids in a closed container with an absorbent dry-pack available from your provider.
- **Schedule Regular and Periodic Checkups with Your Provider:** In-office cleaning and servicing are usually included free with your purchase of hearing aids and you should take advantage of this. We recommend servicing be done at least every

three months (like servicing an expensive car). Hearing aids should be checked for power loss, dirty contact points, plugged vents and openings, and so forth. A more comprehensive servicing should be performed at least annually. This should include electroacoustic analysis (test box evaluation to ensure maintenance of original manufacturer's performance specifications). BTE users should also have the tubing replaced at this time (if not needed at 6 months). There may be a modest charge for this more comprehensive servicing but it's worth it. Residents of drier climates like Arizona will need more frequent tubing changes than those living in more moist environments like Louisiana. Next to daily cleaning, regular in-office servicing is the most important maintenance you can obtain.

Have a Spare Set of Hearing Aids

We conclude with a discussion of hearing aid spares. We hope it's clear from the information contained in this chapter that basic knowledge of hearing aid operation together with use of simple maintenance techniques can go a long way to preventing hearing aid breakdown. We hope it's also apparent that despite your best efforts, without warning, your hearing aids can fail from time to time. If you're a person who's totally dependent on your hearing aids in order to communicate, you might want to consider the purchase of backup hearing aids for use in emergencies. Maintaining two sets of hearing aids may initially cost more. It could be argued, however, that two sets used more or less alternately will last twice as long as one set used full time. So, spare aids may not cost more in the long run. It's kind of like the wisdom of owning two sets of shoes versus only one set. For some users, this works. Also, the availability of spare hearing aids removes the anxiety which might accompany this loss. (Some dispensers provide loaner instruments which may or may not be suitable to your personal needs but is worth inquiring).

How can you judge whether you should have spare hearing aids? The best test we know is an honest answer to the following question: "Does the mere thought of even a temporary loss of the use of your hearing aids create in you the slightest tinge of anxiety?" If it does, then you probably should have a spare set.

Actually, the availability of "spares" is something we all insist upon with commonly used devices we consider vital. (Our cars have spare tires, for example, so we can avoid panicking when a tire fails.) In our experience, people with severe hearing loss will regularly maintain a backup set of hearing aids, especially when the livelihood of such individuals is dependent on good hearing. Furthermore, the federal government for decades has issued to eligible military veterans two complete sets of hearing aids so that good hearing won't be interrupted by temporary breakdowns. You may be one who would also like the extra security of backup instruments in case yours go in for repair. Backup hearing aids can be the still-functioning old set that you just replaced with new ones, or where money is of lesser concern, they can be hearing aids of more current vintage. If you choose to purchase or otherwise have available a set of spare hearing aids, try to ensure that they take the same size battery as your regular ones. This will lend itself to far more convenience than having to store and maintain two different kinds of fresh batteries.

Hearing Aid Disuse and Longevity

The question arises, "Will my spare hearing aids wear out faster or maybe even slower if they're not used regularly?" It's true that peak performance of electromechanical devices can decline with disuse. This need not happen with spare hearing aids, however. This is avoided by rotating them periodically with your regular instruments, for example, once each month or more. This level of activity will keep them going and assure you that they're available and working if and when needed. During extended periods of storage (30 days or longer) the batteries should be completely removed so as to prevent corrosion from possible leakage.

CONCLUSIONS

Today's hearing aids, products of an unprecedented technology, are creations of remarkable quality. Their more accommodating size, improved performance overall and generally high reliability are characteristics as impressive to most audiologists and hearing instrument specialists as they perhaps are to you. They're built to operate for long hours under adverse conditions and they do so with batteries that, while smaller, work harder and produce more energy for their size than those of an earlier era. And for the most part, these hearing instruments perform their valuable service unfailingly.

We hope a thorough understanding of troubleshooting and maintenance principles discussed in this chapter will help you achieve an extended life of service from your hearing aids with a minimum of breakdowns. You deserve no less.

CHAPTER NINE

Ten Questions and Answers:
What the Experts Say

Richard Carmen, Au.D

It isn't possible to address all issues pertaining to hearing loss and hearing aids in a single book. There will always be some questions that remain unanswered in even the most comprehensive approach. With this in mind, I went fishing for probing questions you yourself might ask, and then I searched for the most seasoned professionals to answer them. Here's what evolved, and what the experts say.

1. How can we change present prejudices and misunderstanding about hearing loss and the use of hearing aids?

Ray P. Cuzzort, Ph.D., Boulder, Colorado. Dr. Cuzzort taught sociology at the University of Colorado for the past 30 years. He has written books on social theory and social statistics. His interest in stigmatization goes back to the early 1960s.

The foremost concern with any prosthetic device is how effectively it deals with the physical defect it seeks to correct. This is a relative matter and not as simple as it might first appear to be. If a defect is seriously debilitating, a moderately effective prosthetic device will be relied on. However, if a defect is not seriously stigmatizing, only a superbly effective prosthetic device is likely to be preferred by a user. Complicating the issue is the extent to which revealing the defect is considered stigmatizing by the person involved. If the defect is not seriously stigmatizing, then a prosthetic device is more likely to be used. For example, teenagers wear dental braces despite their mildly disfiguring appearance because ill-formed teeth are not seriously stigmatizing. Wearing a hearing aid, however, suggests that the wearer could be socially handicapped.

People commonly wear glasses when they don't need them. Sunglasses are worn in dark cafes by men and women who want to look "hip." Similarly, "bop" glasses are worn by ghetto youngsters who want to look like jazz musicians. The obvious point being made here is that glasses are not only a prosthetic device, but a stylistic one—a part of one's attire, so to speak. Like any other item of attire, glasses can enhance the image one is trying to project. They can also

159

detract from it.

Another consideration to deal with is the folk history of a prosthetic device and how that history is perceived by the person faced with using the device. What associations does such a history bring to mind? For one thing, glasses are associated with intellectuals, office clerks, and bookish people. These are not strong positive associations, nor are they terribly negative ones either. Glasses don't threaten the image an individual is trying to sustain.

In light of the above comments, we can turn our attention to the hearing aid. Its history, for many people, goes back to a time when a huge, trumpet-like device was waved by a crotchety old person in the direction of someone talking. It was commonly used by women in the advanced stages of senility. Note: this perception does not have to be accurate—it only has to exist in order to have some effect. (For both functional reasons and to rid the hearing aid of this onus, its design has moved quickly toward extremely small and relatively easy-to-hide versions.)

Glasses have no age-specific associations, but hearing aids are seen as an indication of the infirmities that come with being older. In modern America, protests to the contrary, being old is a problem with respect to being stigmatized. It's very likely the case that when an individual is confronted with the choice of being stigmatized by a prosthetic device or being helped by it, avoidance of the stigma will be as important, or more important than the functional value of the device. At the same time, it should also be recognized that stigmatization is a social creation. What is stigmatizing in one social context is not necessarily stigmatizing in another. (The classic example of this is the jagged facial scar that means one thing if it comes from an automobile accident and another if it comes from a duel of honor.) If this is so, then shifting attitudes toward aging as a stigmatizing condition will possibly bring about shifting attitudes toward the use of amplification.

Any campaigns toward changing public perception of hearing aids might consider the following possibilities. First, show more young people, even children, in situations where hearing aids are of benefit. More broadly, show people of varied ages and in different social contexts who are relying on hearing aids. Second, provide specific and compelling measures of the effectiveness of hearing aids. This is a primary concern in any campaign to improve acceptance. Third, direct some attention to the non-hearing aid user. Social interactions, even of a very informal nature, are stressful. If hearing aid users are convinced that people will shun them because they have hearing problems, they will be more likely either to put their hearing aids aside, or avoid people. If hearing aid users can be persuaded that non-hearing aid users are not inclined to perceive them as stigmatized, then hearing aids will be more acceptable.

Fourth, in a modern social context in which a variety of physical handicaps have been granted more tolerant social perceptions, deafness should be defined as a condition that can be effectively dealt with by the use of hearing aids, by sensitivity on the part of all involved with those who are hearing impaired, and by a willingness on the part of the hearing impaired person to remain a participating member of the human community.

2. The title of "Miss America" must be many a young girl's dream. As you know, in earlier years, no one with a disability stood a chance of winning this competition. The fact that you are deaf and won the Crown was something that must have touched the hearts of everyone, especially others with hearing loss. What was one of your most formidable challenges growing up with loss of hearing, and how did you overcome it?

Heather Whitestone McCallum, "Miss America 1995," is now married, and has authored a book about living with loss of hearing: Listening with My Heart (Doubleday, 1997).

My greatest challenge was communication, much like other profoundly deaf children. I often felt frustrated and lonely because I couldn't keep up with the hearing world. I found that I had to repeat the pronunciation of words over and over again until I said them correctly. It took me six years just to correctly say my last name. I grew up, and still live, in the South, and naturally, we southerners have an accent. Unfortunately, accents make it more complicated for me to understand and read lips.

I still have problems with communication. My deafness will always challenge me. I overcome this problem by facing the reality of it. I have to take responsibility by letting people know that I do not correctly hear their words, and that they need to talk more slowly and look at me more so that I can read their lips. On occasion, I've even had some people write down what they said. Most of the time I communicate well because for more than 20 years I have communicated with, and lived among "hearing people." I believe that the more communication deaf and hard of hearing people have with the hearing world, the better they will master their problems. The problem will never go away. But they can improve situations between the hearing world and themselves by using creative ideas.

3. **All of us who dispense hearing aids hear from many users that they feel they've spent a lot of money, and in some cases, too much money. Since the early 1970s, the standard in-the-ear (ITE) hearing instrument has not only doubled, tripled, but in some cases, four- and five-folded in cost to the consumer. What do you say to someone asking for an explanation of what appears, at least on the surface, to be unfairly escalating prices?**

Michele D. Hartlove, MA., is Acting Executive Director of the Better Hearing Institute, Washington, D.C. Ms. Hartlove has been with BHI for 14 years. She is past Chairman of the Council for Better Hearing and Speech Month.

It's indisputable that the cost of a hearing aid to the consumer has escalated dramatically in comparison to what it was in the 1970s. But so have most things, including basic necessities. For example, you can spend $3.50 today and get a premium loaf of bread that contains up to twelve—and perhaps even more—grains. It can be low in both sodium and cholesterol. The consumer can choose not only how the grains are ground but the type of oven used to bake it. Keep in mind that this kind of baking wasn't available 20 years ago when the typical loaf was 35 cents.

Today, hearing aids can do much more than what they could do two decades ago. For $350 in the 1970s, a consumer could buy an ITE which amplified all sounds. Background noise and conversations were transmitted on an equal decibel level. Appearance was secondary, and large ITEs with knobs, controls, or wires were the rule rather than the exception.

Today, a highly priced hearing aid is the product of the latest technology. Some ITEs are virtually invisible. Many hearing aids no longer require knobs and controls because the instruments automatically adjust sound quality. Different hearing capabilities are available through the push of a button, such as with programmable systems which are wireless and remotely controlled. Some circuits in hearing aids can even automatically adjust to sound levels in the environment. And today's hearing instruments provide balanced sound in different listening environments such as in the office, at home, on the telephone, or at a concert.

So a loaf of bread, although the staff of life, is still just a loaf of bread. But today's hearing aids are the key to vital and rewarding communication which is of incalculable value.

4. **Once consumers have made the decision to obtain hearing aids, and yet before they make their first visit to a hearing health care professional, they have certain expectations. While many people are hopeful of the outcome and look forward to renewed hearing, others are unduly influenced by something negative in the press, or by people they know who have unsuccessfully tried hearing aids. How can these consumers best temper the unfortunate experiences of others?**

Mary Caccavo, Ph.D., is current President of the Academy of Dispensing Audiologists, herself an Audiologist who has been dispensing hearing aids for many years. She has served on the Board of the Indiana Academy of Audiology and on the Indiana licensing Board.

If you listen to reports of unsuccessful hearing aid trials by others, you should be aware that you may not be getting the whole story. For example, it's common practice for hearing health care professionals to recommend a hearing aid for each impaired ear. Some patients ask, "Can't I *just get by* with one?" If one hearing aid is chosen when two are indicated, you'll most likely find your ability to understand speech in noise to be unsatisfactory and complain that the instrument did not perform to your level of satisfaction. In reality, you get what you requested because one hearing aid *barely allows you to get by!*

Each person with hearing loss is different and unique. Adjusting to hearing aids and learning to retrain your brain to understand speech in environments which used to be impossible take time and in many cases a rehabilitation plan. This is why it's so important to trust your own experience—not someone else's. Your professional will design a hearing aid evaluation program for your hearing needs which complements your lifestyle. In many cases, keeping a journal of your daily activities and where you notice an improvement in communication will help you track your progress and the need for adjustments. Your positive attitude and willingness to follow through with appointments for adjustments is an important part of the rehabilitative process.

5. **Is there a problem in the United States regarding the unintentional swallowing of hearing aid batteries, and if so, what consumer protection would you recommend?**

Rose Ann G. Soloway, RN, is a board-certified clinical toxicologist with the National Capitol Poison Center. She is also Administrator of the American Association of Poison Control Centers. The National Button Ingestion Hotline Telephone Number is 212-625-3333 (collect if necessary).

It's hard to imagine swallowing a hearing aid battery, but it happens more than 1,000 times each year. And it's easier than you might think. Since Toby Litovitz, M.D. established the National Button Battery Ingestion Hotline and Registry in 1982, she and the Hotline staff have managed more than 6,000 cases of battery ingestions. It occurs in children and adults.

Children swallow hearing aid batteries for the same reasons they swallow other things within reach. They're curious, they explore everything within reach, and anything can end up in the mouth. They swallow batteries pried from their own hearing aids or their family member's hearing aids, or those that may be merely left on tables or in drawers. They also have been known to locate them in the trash. But hearing aids are only one source of this problem for children. They'll swallow batteries from toys, cameras, calculators, jewelry and so forth. Protection is available by using child-resistant hearing aids and by keeping batteries in their original packaging, stored out of children's reach. To dispose of batteries, wrap them securely in something before discarding, so they can't be easily retrieved.

Adults are apt to swallow batteries by mistaking them for pills. Sometimes, they're put in the same pockets as pills. People think they're swallowing pills but are later surprised to find pills, and no batteries in their pocket! A similar mistake occurs when loose batteries are stored in old pill bottles. Adults who mistakenly think they can test a battery's charge by placing it on the tongue also wind up swallowing a tiny, slippery battery. The same thing happens to adults who put them in their mouths to keep them handy while they change batteries.

While it's unusual for swallowed batteries to cause harm, injury and death have occurred in a few cases. Most of the time, a swallowed battery passes through the esophagus and into the stomach. Gradually, it works its way through the intestinal tract and is eliminated in the stool. Rarely, the battery gets stuck in the esophagus. This situation doesn't always cause symptoms right away, but is very dangerous because it can cause a lot of bleeding. Also rarely, a battery that passes through the esophagus and stomach later gets stuck somewhere in the intestinal tract.

If someone swallows a battery, immediately call the 24-hour National Button Battery Ingestion Hotline at 202-625-3333. You may call collect. You may also call your physician or local poison center, and ask them to call the Battery Hotline. The nurses at the Hotline will ask you to have a chest x-ray immediately. If it shows that the battery has passed through the esophagus into the stomach, nothing needs to be done—or should be done—except watching and waiting for its passage. In young children, this could occur in just a day or two; in elderly people, such passage could take two or even three months. If the battery hasn't been seen within a week, another x-ray will usually be recommended to be sure it is moving. The Hotline staff will stay in touch with you until the battery has passed, then ask you to mail it in for evaluation. Of course, if you develop any symptoms, the Hotline nurses will work with your physician to decide if any treatment is necessary.

Keep in mind that it is rarely necessary for surgery to be done! Be sure to contact the Battery Hotline immediately if someone suggests surgery to remove a battery.

6. Under what circumstances should people be concerned enough about their hearing disorder to be seen medically by a family physician, otologist or otolaryngologist?

Charles Krause, MD is President of the American Academy of Otolaryngology—Head and Neck Surgery, and Professor at the University of Michigan. He has taught internationally, has more than 100 scholarly publications to his credit, and serves on five editorial boards.

Many individuals notice a problem with their ears, and wonder whether they should see a physician before being evaluated for hearing aids. Though no guidelines are correct for every circumstance, the following situations should be reason for evaluation by an ear, nose and throat specialist (otologist or otolaryngologist). These conditions are essentially what the Food and Drug Administration recommend that your hearing instrument specialist or audiologist consider prior to considering you for hearing aids:

a) *A visible congenital or traumatic deformity of the ear.* Many of these are accompanied by hearing loss, and most can be improved both functionally and in appearance.

b) *A history of active drainage from the ear,* particularly if it's foul smelling. Except for earwax, most drainage from an ear is caused by active infection. Left untreated, the infection can cause permanent damage.

c) *A history of sudden or rapidly progressive hearing loss.* Except when caused by a plug of earwax, a sudden loss of hearing needs careful evaluation, especially if it occurs in one ear.

d) *Active dizziness,* particularly "spinning," is caused by a problem in the inner ear, and may be associated with a hearing loss.

e) *A conductive hearing loss* (air-bone gap on audiometric testing) of at least 15 dB in the primary hearing frequencies. Such a hearing loss can usually be restored with medical treatment.

f) *Pain or discomfort in an ear.* This is usually caused by infection in the external or middle ear. Medical evaluation and treatment usually result in rapid resolution of the pain.

g) *Visible evidence of a plug of earwax or foreign body in the ear canal.* Such an obstruction is best removed using careful extraction rather than irrigation.

By applying these guidelines, you'll have a more informed idea of when a medical specialty evaluation is necessary.

7. **Most people have heard of the condition of Meniere's Disease, but few, including those suffering from it, have a good understanding of the problem. Can you help clarify this disorder, and how it might differ from the similar condition of labyrinthitis?**

Dennis Poe, M.D., of Massachusettes Eye and Ear, Boston, is an otolaryngologist specializing in neurotologic surgery and is a Board Member of the Meniere's Society. He is considered a foremost expert on Meniere's Disease and is actively involved in Meniere's research.

Dizziness and balance disorders are very common and rank among the most frequent problems seen on a daily basis by health care providers of all types. Labyrinthitis, an inflammation or irritation of the inner ear, and Meniere's Disease, a disruption of the inner ear due to fluid swelling, are the two most common inner ear disturbances that cause the sudden onset of vertigo or imbalance, and both may be associated with varying degrees of hearing loss. Medical professionals define vertigo as *any hallucination of movement when in fact no real movement has occurred.* The most common form of this is the spinning sensation that results after rapidly rotating oneself and stopping quickly. If vertigo is severe enough, it can cause secondary symptoms of nausea, vomiting, and cold sweats. It's estimated that about one third of the population will experience a significant bout of sudden vertigo during their lifetime, and the vast majority of these are due to labyrinthitis. Still, Meniere's is common enough to affect as many as one out of 50 individuals.

Labyrinthitis is presumably often caused by viral inflammation of the vestibular (balance) organ causing vertigo and balance disturbances without hearing loss, but more severe cases may also damage hearing. Severe cases can cause sudden unexpected vertiginous attacks with a complete loss of balance that is made worse by any head movements or by watching anything move. These symptoms can often last for hours causing nausea, vomiting, sometimes diarrhea, all of which can be a profoundly frightening experience. The episodes are usually quite harmless and completely resolve on their own in a few days without any treatment. Like many viral illnesses, it normally will not recur. More severe forms may cause a few "after shock" spells of lesser magnitude within a few days of the original attack. Once the acute vertigo attacks have subsided, there's a period of dysequilibrium—a sensation that the balance is off, and may last for hours, days, or many weeks, depending on the severity of the attacks. Treatment is usually limited to symptom relief with medications to quiet the balance system. A regular exercise program is recommended to speed up the compensation process after the balance injury.

Meniere's Disease is believed to be the long-term result of an injury to the labyrinth, such as severe labyrinthitis, that has failed to heal properly and has gone on to become a recurring cause of vertigo attacks and hearing injury.

The symptoms of Meniere's Disease (recurring vertigo attacks, fluctuating hearing loss, abnormal noises in the ear—tinnitus—and pressure or fullness in the ear) are caused by a condition known as endolymphatic hydrops (swelling of the endolymph). This is the fluid that fills the innermost compartment of the inner ear. The excessive pressure is believed to result from a breakdown in the pressure-regulating mechanisms and can be simplistically likened to water on the knee years after an injury. When the inner ear fluids swell, it causes some strain which initially may be mistaken for pressure in the middle ear, as might be experienced with infections, or airplane travel. If the swelling continues, hearing loss, especially in the lower frequencies, may fluctuate and be associated with tinnitus, the warning noises the ear creates when injured.

Ultimately, unprovoked episodes of spinning vertigo can develop, sometimes even waking someone from sleep with a violent sense of rotation, nausea, and vomiting. The attack can last for minutes or hours and usually subsides, leaving the person exhausted and very unstable with significant dysequilibrium for many more hours, days, or even weeks, going through the same vestibular compensation recovery as occurs after a labyrinthitis spell.

Meniere's is much more disabling because these spells recur unexpectedly and with variable frequency, creating a tremendous loss of confidence in oneself. If the vertigo attacks occur frequently enough, there may be insufficient time between spells for vestibular compensation to occur and the person will experience chronic dysequilibrium with intermittent vertigo attacks, never having a chance to fully recover. Health care professionals and patients have difficulty sorting out the difference between spontaneous vertigo attacks, and the head movement or position-induced vertigo and dysequilibrium during the compensation phase.

In its early stages, Meniere's Disease can be exceedingly difficult to diagnose but early recognition and treatment may be useful in arresting the progression of the disease from its natural course of hearing and balance degeneration. Each time a hydrops (accumulation of fluid) episode occurs, it does a small amount of cumulative but permanent damage to the inner ear.

Treatment for Meniere's Disease is directed toward controlling the endolymphatic fluid swelling since in 90 percent of patients, no active cause will be identified. The body uses sodium as its principal regulator of fluid balance, so a strict 2000 milligram daily sodium-restricted diet is recommended. A sodium guidebook is recommended to learn about packaging labels and natural sodium content in foods. Simply removing the salt shaker from the table is inadequate to treat this disorder and strict regular adherence to a 2000 mg diet is strongly recommended. Most people who do adhere to their diet notice a substantial difference when they eat out and cannot control their sodium intake, experiencing more symptoms within one or two days afterwards.

The second most important factor in controlling Meniere's is controlling stress. The hormonal release associated with stress has a profound effect on aggravating Meniere's Disease, although, the mechanism for this is poorly understood. It's quite obvious that an increase in spells occurs during times of crises, injury, or illness. Gaining emotional control over Meniere's Disease is a critical issue in preventing oneself falling into the trap of becoming a victim to the condition. Victims live in the constant fear that an attack may occur, and the very stress of this fear actually creates more attacks. Many

168

people who understand this situation find that they can exert their will over spells, and sometimes avert them. Caffeine, nicotine, and other powerful stimulants have also been known to aggravate Meniere's. Decaffeinated beverages and cessation of smoking are always recommended.

Physicians will often add a diuretic (water pill) to the treatment regimen to reduce the inner ear fluid pressure. Diuretics are often used for several months, then discontinued if the condition can be controlled by diet alone. If the spells cannot be adequately managed, then vestibular suppressants are often prescribed. These medications are all central nervous system depressants in nature, trying to slow down the abnormal impulses within the balance system, or anti-nausea medications which also help stabilize balance. Such medications are for symptom assistance only and do not prevent vertigo attacks. They may be used on a daily, even round-the-clock basis for short periods of time.

Medical treatment for Meniere's is generally successful in controlling the attacks, limiting them to one or two significant attacks per year, and most people don't require surgery. About 20 percent of Meniere's patients ultimately fail medical treatment and desire surgical intervention to stop the vertiginous attacks. Most of the procedures are designed to deaden the affected balance nerve so that the abnormal imbalance signals no longer reach the brain, and the vertigo attacks cease. When there are no further disturbances in the balance system, vestibular compensation can occur as the opposite inner ear adjusts to the new balance arrangement.

8. We know that the heart carries nutrition throughout the body, including the ear. Without absorption of nutrients critical to hearing, its function would stop. For example, many people who have gone on a starvation diet as a political protest have lost some of their hearing. Since we've become so vitamin and mineral conscious, is there anything you might recommend which has been shown to positively impact the hearing mechanism?

Martin Dayton, D.O., is current Chairman of the Board of the International and American Association of Clinical Nutritionists. He is Board certified, well-published in his field, and has a clinical practice in Miami Beach. Also, he is an Assistant Clinical Professor at Nova Southeastern University, College of Osteopathic Medicine.

Unfortunately, no specific nutritional treatment is generally used or known to address hearing loss in all people. However, strategies do exist which may address the needs of the individual with impaired hearing, in accordance with the unique circumstances of the person. These circumstances are governed by the inherited and acquired strengths and weaknesses of the individual and the conditions under which the person exists.

A child may have an inherited predisposition to allergies and live in an environment where junk food is a staple. This child may be prone to develop a form of "stuffed ears" known as serous otitis media. Fluid accumulates in the middle ear due to allergy-mediated inflammation, swelling, and closure of the eustachian tube. Dysfunctional pressures may develop in the ear. Infection may take hold in part due to impaired transport of immune factors to the area and impaired drainage of toxic fluids from the ear due to swelling.

On the other hand, an elderly person with an inherited predisposition to hardening of the arteries who eats the nutritionally sub-optimal standard American diet may develop progressive hearing loss. This is due to auditory nerve tissue deterioration associated with impaired circulation—accelerated with aging. Perhaps, accumulation of environmental or pharmaceutical toxic materials with time is also a role in the manifestation of hearing loss.

These two cases illustrate how diverse the contributing circumstances can be in regard to the manifestation of hearing loss. Each case must be handled differently in the use of nutrition to address the same goal of improved hearing. The child in the first example needs to avoid foods which may trigger allergies. Wheat, cow's milk, peanuts, chocolate, eggs, and soy are frequent offenders. Various methods are used to determine which foods need to be avoided, when and how often. Various methods may be used to reduce such sensitivities. Plant extracts from stinging nettles, aloe vera, citrus and seeds of grapes may reverse the allergic processes. Vitamins, such as C and pantothenic acid may also be useful. Addressing deficiencies of various substances improves overall resistance to disease.

The older person in the second example needs to improve circulation and, in part, to reverse processes which lead to deterioration. Plant extracts such as ginko biloba improves efficiency and function of tissues subject to sub-optimal circulation. Niacin increases blood flow via dilation of blood vessels and may restore cholesterol to a more optimal state. Turmeric (Curcuma longa) reduces the tendency to build-up of blockages within the walls of arteries, and helps prevent deterioration of tissues. Various substances help prevent tissue deterioration and foster repair. Optimal repair of nerve tissue needs an abundance of the components found in such tissue cofactors which make them work. Lecithin contains materials needed for cell wall repair, and chemicals needed for communication between nerve cells. Vitamin B12, alpha-lipoic acid, and thiamin are co-factors which help maintain and repair nerve tissue. Various nutritional substances help to directly remove toxins, or fortify the detoxification organs of the body so they are more effective in achieving their intended purpose. Adequate detoxification is necessary for normal function and repair. Vitamin C, garlic, and chlorella, are helpful. And many nutritional substances have multiple benefits.

The most important aspect of nutritional care in regard to ear problems lies between the ears in taking care of the needs of the rest of the person who is attached to the ears.

9. I suspect that among most people, there's a great misunderstanding of what a cochlear implant is. I've seen many patients over the years (who do well with standard hearing aids) asking me if I think they're candidates for this surgery. Can you offer some clarity on what a cochlear implant is, who really is a candidate, and what promise does the future hold for such implantation in milder losses of hearing?

William Luxford, M.D. has been performing cochlear implant surgeries for many years. He is extensively published in this area, and is an associate of the House Ear Institute in Los Angeles.

In general, cochlear implant candidates have a bilateral profound sensorineural hearing loss, receive little or no benefit from conventional hearing aids, are in good physical and mental health, and have the motivation and patience to complete a rehabilitation program. A cochlear implant is an electronic prosthetic device that is surgically placed in the inner ear, under the skin behind the ear to provide sound perception to selected severe-to-profound hearing impaired individuals. In addition to the internal component of the system, the cochlear implant has external parts that are worn outside the ear, including the microphone, speech processor, headpiece antenna and cable. A cochlear implant is NOT a hearing aid (See Figure 9-1). A hearing aid amplifies acoustic signals, thereby making sounds louder and clearer to the hearing impaired person. Hearing aid-amplified acoustic signals are delivered to the ear and converted into electrical impulses by the hair cells of the inner ear in exactly the same manner as sounds that are transmitted to the normal hearing ear. A cochlear implant, on the other hand, converts acoustic sound vibrations into electrical signals, which are then coded and patterned in a manner designed to enhance speech perception. Through an externally worn antenna and internally implanted receiver, these coded electrical signals are then transmitted to an electrode in the inner ear which directly stimulates the auditory nerve fibers, thus bypassing the damaged hair cells of the cochlea. The electrical impulses are delivered to the brain where they are interpreted as meaningful sounds.

Potential candidates for cochlear implants include both children and adults with a wide age range. For the most part, children are at least 18 months old, while there are many people in their 80s who are successful users. Candidates undergo a very thorough evaluation, including medical, audiological and radiological assessment. The medical evaluation includes a complete history and physical examination to detect problems that might interfere with the patient's ability to complete either the surgical or rehabilitative measures of implantation. In adults, the cause of deafness would not seem as important as its onset. Adults who become deaf later in life, and who have fully developed speech and language before losing their hearing,

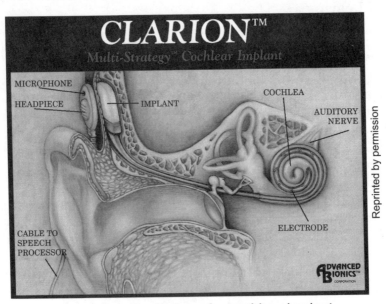

Figure 9-1: Illustration of a cochlear implant.

COCHLEA

are able to make better use of the implant than those who are born deaf or lose their hearing very early in life. On the other hand, the prelingually deafened child, if implanted early in life, can receive a great deal of benefit from a cochlear implant.

Counseling is important so that the patient and the family will have realistic expectations regarding benefits and limitations. Support from family and friends is essential in the rehabilitative process. The definition of success is different from person to person, and family to family. Memory of sound appears to be one of the most important factors for success in adults. Early implantation, and placement in an educational program that emphasizes development of auditory skills appear to be important factors for success in children.

Initially, only those patients who were stone deaf in both ears were considered implant candidates. With significant improvements in implant technology and signal processing, the benefits gained by implanted patients, both children and adults, have markedly improved. These improvements have led to a broadening of the criteria for implant patients. Selected patients with severe hearing loss receiving some benefit from appropriately fitted hearing aids, are now considered possible implant candidates. Hearing aid technology has also improved. Most likely, patients with mild and moderate hearing loss will be candidates for hearing aids. Patients with severe loss will be candidates for either a hearing aid or cochlear implant, depending upon how well they function with the appropriate device. Patients with profound hearing loss will probably receive the best benefit through the use of a cochlear implant.

10. It would seem that one of the final frontiers in human research on impaired hearing would be to establish methods of regenerating inner ear hair cells. As most of us would *assume*, once hair cells die, it results in permanent and irreversible sensorineural hearing loss. Would you share with readers what you've discovered, and any implications it might hold for restoration of hearing in humans?

Edwin W Rubel, Ph.D., is Virginia Merrill Bloedel Professor of Hearing Science, and Professor in the Departments of Otolaryngology—Head and Neck Surgery, Physiology/Biophysics, Neurological Surgery and Psychology at the University of Washington. He has published over 200 scientific articles and edited three books on various topics related to development and plasticity of the auditory system.

The first point I'd like to make is that research on hair cell regeneration was not a major topic of research in hearing science until 1986-87. At that time, my group was one of two that discovered mature birds had the remarkable natural ability to reform their inner ear hair cells after either damage produced by loud noises, or after damage produced by certain therapeutic drugs like antibiotics (See Figure 9-2). This was quite startling to us as well as to the rest of the scientific community. Confirmation through DNA technology supported what we were seeing. After damage occurred, there were indeed new hair cells generated by renewed cell division in several species of fully mature birds.

The work on mammals now is at a point where we can induce a small amount of cell division in the inner ear in a dish (that is, in culture), as well as in vivo (occurring within a living organism). This has been done in mice, guinea pigs and rats using a variety of growth-promoting molecules. Therefore, we at least know that it's possible to induce the first stage in the inner ear sensory epithelium of mature mammals. The sensory epithelium make up parts of the cochlea that cause the initial response to sound. So far, hair cell regeneration has only been done in the balance parts of the inner ear, but we're working on the cochlea.

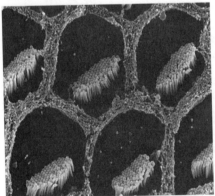 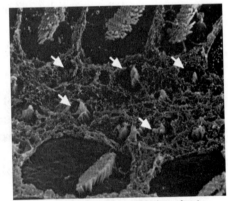

Figure 9-2: Left photo shows normal hair cell clusters. Right photo arrows show hair cell regeneration after being destroyed.

The good news is that for the first time in history, there are teams of investigators worldwide exploring the possibility that hair cell regeneration can be induced in the mammal and human cochlea. Eight years ago there were only two laboratories exploring this possibility. Now there are probably 20 or 30. The bad news is funding.

It's a real problem. Until we actually find candidate molecules for use in humans, this research won't be taken over by pharmaceutical companies. Once they step in, they will heavily invest in developing human therapies. But, until then, the entire cost of this research must be borne by the federal government and private foundations. I feel that within 5 to 10 years, we'll find out if it's possible to regenerate hair cells at robust levels, that is, sufficient to restore hearing in mammals. From there, it could be as little as another 10 years until we achieve hair cell regeneration in humans. If successful, it could eliminate some of the need for hearing aids and cochlear implants as we now know them.

When I started this work, somebody said to me that I'd never be able to restore the complexity and intricacies of hair cells in humans or other mammals. My response hasn't changed: you could be right, but without trying, it surely won't happen. If our goal is to actually restore hearing—it's the only game in town.

Introduction

Section III: Management of Hearing Loss

Robin L. Holm, BC-HIS
Senior Editor, *Audecibel*
Executive Director, International Hearing Society
Livonia, Michigan

This section is a *must read* for everyone who either is experiencing communication failures due to impaired hearing, or who is the loved one of a hard of hearing person. You will learn from the firsthand experience of the author, practical skills you can begin using today and every day for the rest of your life.

You are now well on the road to communication rehabilitation. You have faced your hearing loss head on; wearing a hearing instrument has become a way of life. Hearing aids are not the only answer. They are, in fact, just one piece of a very complex puzzle.

In Chapter 10, Dr. Ross, who's been wearing hearing aids since 1952, shares his strategies for living in a world designed for hearing people. He teaches you how to view communication issues, and shows you how to adopt new and different strategies that <u>will</u> make a difference in how well you interact with others. Remember, you are not alone. Your expectations play a key role in your success.

In the next chapter, Dr. Tyler discusses tinnitus, more commonly described as ringing in the ears, which affects millions of people. While there is no *consistent* effective treatment for tinnitus, the author discusses a variety of treatment options, some more effective than others, depending on your individual situation. His observations on stress, diet and lifestyle are particularly informative even for those who do not suffer from this often debilitating condition.

In the final chapter of this section, Dr Campbell cites an old *ism*, "An ounce of prevention is worth a pound of cure." No truer statement can be made about hearing loss. Besides aging as a factor, one of the most common causes of hearing loss is noise. Who's really at risk? As you'll discover, virtually everyone! Hearing can be impaired by everything from a household vacuum cleaner, to a fire engine, to a jet engine or rock concert. We live in a noisy world. The author will show you how to protect yourself, and your loved ones, from additional hearing loss caused by noise.

Equally important is her discussion on ototoxic medications; that is, those drugs known to damage hearing. Aspirin, certain antibiotics, and some cancer-fighting chemicals are all on the list. Be an informed consumer. This chapter will offer you the knowledge and tools necessary to discuss your situation with your primary care physician.

Breaking through the communication barrier is an everyday process. Each day you'll develop new skills to enhance your current communication abilities, and to protect yourself from further risk of continued impairment. The pearls of wisdom you harvest from this section could last a lifetime.

CHAPTER TEN

Ways to Improve Listening and Hearing

Mark Ross, Ph.D.

Dr. Ross received his Doctorate at Stanford University. He has worked as a Clinical Audiologist, a Director of a School for the Deaf, Director of Research and Training at the League for the Hard of Hearing, and as a Professor of Audiology at the University of Connecticut where he's now an Emeritus Professor of Audiology. Currently, Dr. Ross is an Associate at the Rehabilitation Engineering Resource Center (RERC) at the Lexington Center in Jackson Heights, N.Y. Among his activities for the RERC is a bimonthly feature that he writes on Developments in Research and Technology for *Hearing Loss: the Journal of Self Help for Hard of Hearing People*.

This chapter will be presented in several major sections. I'll begin by discussing your responsibilities in communicating, then your initial experiences to hearing aids. While this topic has been covered in other sections of the book, my focus here is how you learn to interpret and enjoy the new world of sound to which you've suddenly been exposed. I'll follow this by discussing speechreading and various exercises that will help you make the most of your residual hearing. Finally, in the last section, I'll present some "hearing tactics," that is, various kinds of adaptations to real-life situations that can help you increase your communication abilities. All of these I've had occasion to personally practice in the many years I've worn hearing aids.

I don't know any hard of hearing person who, if a magic wand were available that could be used to wave away his or her hearing loss, would not jump at this miraculous cure. I know that I would like to be at the head of the line! But life is not a fairy tale and magic wands are in short supply. For most of us with hearing loss, it's simply a pain, one whose impact we're constantly trying to overcome or minimize. We don't approach the world as "hard of hearing" people, seeking acceptance as a separate social entity. On the contrary, by striving to reduce the impact of hearing loss in our lives, we're trying *not* to make it a defining condition of our personal identity. To realize our goal of continued engagement with the larger society—with our friends, family, jobs, and interests—we employ the modern technology of hearing aids and other assistive devices. And we use various communication strategies to overcome and reduce the inevitable consequences of hearing loss.

By "communication strategies" I mean any activity that might increase your ability to understand speech, either generally or in particular situations. I don't mean technological solutions. These are crucial prerequisite considerations, but the adjustment process doesn't end there. There are other things you can do to improve your functional communication. When you purchased hearing aids or some other assistive device, you depended upon the hearing health care provider's expertise to help make the proper decision. When it comes to communication strategies and making the best use of your hearing aids, you have to take the major responsibility for your own actions. The concept of personal responsibility for one's own action underlies three recurring themes implicit throughout this chapter (and in other parts of this book), beginning with acknowledgment.

Acknowledgment

The first and indispensable step in practicing effective communication strategies is to accept the reality of the hearing loss. Unless and until you can acknowledge its presence, openly and in a matter of fact way, you are always going to be limited in how effectively you can deal with it. A hearing loss is not something to be ashamed of; it's not a stigma that has to be hidden; <u>its presence does not diminish you as a human being</u>. By denying or projecting your hearing difficulties onto other people's mouths ("people don't talk as clearly as they used to when I was young!"), you fool only yourself. The point is worth emphasizing: the hearing loss is there; magical thinking, denial, not "wanting to talk about it," will not make it go away. If you don't face up to this reality, unpleasant as it may be, you're condemning yourself to a life of unnecessary stress, isolation, and anxiety. Some people will go to almost any length to deny a hearing loss, to themselves and to others. The pity of this attitude, of course, is that while they may try to deny the presence of a hearing loss, they cannot disguise its effects. They still miss and misunderstand everyday conversation, their social and cultural activities gradually diminish, with feelings of stress and anxiety part of their daily fare. As a result, their lives become more and more constricted and less and less satisfying. And if this changing pattern of personal behavior cannot be ascribed to a hearing loss, other conclusions will be drawn, especially by one's family, social circle or co-workers mistaking the problem for early senility, personality changes, or worse. Which is preferable? Having people think you're deliberately ignoring them or letting them know you have a hearing loss and that you're doing something about it? Once you accept yourself, and presumably you're on that road or you wouldn't be reading this book, then the acceptance of others will naturally fall into place.

Assertiveness

"Letting them know" is another way of expressing the second recurring theme in this chapter. Once you've acknowledged the hearing loss, to yourself and to others, you are then in a position to *assert* your communication needs in various kinds of situations. "Assertiveness" is a concept that underlies many of the specific steps I'll be suggesting later. As the person with a hearing loss, you must be willing to inform and educate others about what *they* have to do in order to make it easier for you to understand. It may be as simple as asking the waiter in a restaurant to turn down the background music or to provide you with a written choice of the day's selections, or as involved as arranging the seats at a meeting or suggesting how your conversational partner can be a more effective communicator.

Being more assertive about one's listening needs, asking other folks to modify their behavior, does not come naturally for many people. It may mean changing the habits of a lifetime but it can be done and it can be quite liberating (there's got to be *some* advantage to getting older!). Of course, we don't have to take giant steps in the beginning. Even little ones, as long as we take enough of them, will eventually get us to our goal. And we can be assertive about listening needs without being aggressive or hostile. "Would you mind talking a little louder? I have a hearing loss and that will make it easier for me to understand you," will get better results than, "For Pete's sake, get the mud out of your mouth when you speak to me!" When we assert our hearing needs, we're saying to somebody that, yes, we really do want to communicate with you.

Communication Exchange

And this brings up the third recurring theme in this chapter: both you and the person with whom you are talking are equally involved in a communication exchange. This person wants to be understood as much as you want to understand. Unlike a monologue, conversation is a two-way street. When you suggest that a seating arrangement be modified, or you inform your conversational partners what verbal modifications to make so that you can understand them, it's as much for their benefit as it is for yours. What I'm suggesting is that when you work with and help other people communicate more effectively with you, both you and the other party benefit. So acknowledge your hearing loss, be assertive about your hearing needs, and know that you are a crucial half of any communication interchange.

Getting the Most Out of Your Hearing Aid

As a hard of hearing person, you want to ensure that you're making the most use of your residual hearing, which means maximizing benefit from amplified sound you're receiving through your hearing aids. Indeed, the reason you're reading this book is because you or a loved one has a hearing loss which is causing communication failures: *amplification is the only "therapy" that directly addresses a solution for communication breakdowns.* It's the only measure you can take that directly increases the actual amount of acoustic information available. All the training and practice procedures that are to be covered are predicated on you getting as much useful acoustic information as possible through your hearing aids. Although you should realize some immediate benefit from hearing aids, you should obtain even more help after you are used to them. Getting the most from your hearing aids requires us to consider both some general principles and specific training procedures.

General Principles

Tenacity

First of all, don't get discouraged—and that's second and third of all too. Remember that while you've had a hearing loss for a number of years and have experienced abnormal auditory sensations, for you the sounds you have been receiving are perfectly "normal" (though, of course, they haven't been). Now you're suddenly exposed to not only louder sounds but to a different pattern of sounds.

Patience

You're going to have to reeducate your brain to accept different sound patterns as "normal." As a rather simple analogy, what you're now perceiving with hearing aids can be likened to someone talking English with a very different accent. Just as it takes some time to get used to, for example, a Scotsman speaking English, or for a New Englander to comprehend the speech of someone who comes from the deep south (and vice versa), so will it take some time for you to adjust to the amplified "accent" coming through your hearing aids.

The Adjustment Process

What will happen is that when you first put on your hearing aids on, you're suddenly going to hear many sounds of which you were previously unaware. Many of these sounds will jog familiar memories. For others, you're going to have to consciously identify the source of the sound, either by asking someone or by seeking it out yourself. One woman in a recent hearing aid orientation group was going a little crazy with the hissing and splattering sounds she kept hearing until she realized it was coming from her frying pan. She hadn't heard the sounds of frying food for many years.

All at once you're going to be exposed to a world of sound you forgot existed, such as the whirl of the dishwasher, the whine of an electric can opener, the sounds of birds singing, or the "ting" of your microwave when the food is done. Other familiar sounds will be experienced somewhat differently and may even be disturbing, such as traffic noises in the city, the tumult in your favorite restaurant, and the screeching from your grandchildren's boombox (I'm told it's music). It's true that it's a noisy world in which we live, and it seems to be getting noisier all the time. But it's the only world we have and it's the one in which you're going to feel more comfortable when you can more fully hear what's going on.

Expectations

Not everybody will be able to realize the same degree of benefit from hearing aids. After resisting the notion of hearing aids for years, some people, when they finally relent, expect that hearing aids will re-create their hearing abilities of 50 years ago. It doesn't work that way. While hearing aids will help most people with hearing loss, no matter how advanced a hearing aid, or how skilled the audiologist or hearing instrument specialist, the ultimate benefits achievable through amplification is set by the nature of the hearing loss. Just because Uncle Joe is doing beautifully with hearing aids doesn't mean that Aunt Tilly will do as well, even if they're using the same hearing aids, have the same hearing loss, and work with the same professionals. This means, then, while just about everybody with a hearing loss can obtain *some* benefit from hearing aids, the degree of benefit will vary among individuals. Your satisfaction with hearing aids, therefore, is going to depend greatly on your expectations, which should be set neither too high nor too low.

One important way to develop realistic expectations is to educate yourself about hearing loss (which is what you're doing by reading this book). Another is by talking to other people with hearing loss. And a third is by working closely with the professional who fit you with hearing aids. You'll find most of them ready and willing to help you understand what you can and cannot readily achieve with hearing aids.

Initial Experiences

Every hearing professional seems to have a favorite "recipe" for helping a new user adjust to the new world of sound produced by hearing aids. The user information booklet that comes with your hearing aids undoubtedly contains such material. I really haven't seen any wrong recipes. If you persist and work with your provider, I have no doubt that you'll eventually find your hearing aids helpful. Some professionals suggest that you begin by wearing hearing aids an hour or so each day, gradually increasing the time; others recommend beginning with easy listening situations (such as in quiet while talking to one person) and work yourself up to more difficult listening environments. Still others make recommendations that are basically variations of these two themes. There's nothing wrong with these recipes—they'll work if you try them diligently. *But remember, it's your hearing experiences, and you can modify any rule for your convenience and comfort.*

I have a friend who telephoned me recently, very upset. He had just put on his first set of binaural hearing aids a few days before and was thrilled. His audiologist told him to wear the instruments just an hour each day for the first week and then gradually increase the time in subsequent weeks. Generally, this recommendation does work well for most people. My friend, however, liked the hearing aids. His wife was delighted that she didn't have to yell at him, but pursuant to his audiologist's instructions, he felt he had to take them off after an hour—and strain to hear his favorite television programs! "Can't I wear them more often?" he asked me. In this instance, the general "rule" did not apply. When I told him he could wear them as long as he wanted, he was tremendously relieved.

Be in Control

What I suggest you do is wear your hearing aids for as long each day as you feel comfortable, with the goal of wearing them all day every day. But you have to be satisfied that they're helping you hear better and that they don't hurt your ears after a few hours. Sometimes, depending upon the nature of what you're hearing, you may want to remove them (e.g. at a hard rock concert, mowing the lawn on a windy way, etc.). Go ahead and take them out and don't feel guilty. Remember, you're the boss, they're your ears, your hearing aids, and you're in control. But, you must continue to work closely with the professionals from whom you received the hearing instruments. They can't give you full benefits of their knowledge and experience unless, particularly in the period right after you receive them, you call upon your provider with your questions, comments, and experiences.

Reeducating the Brain

What "getting used to hearing aids" really means is that you'll be undergoing a learning process. Not only will you have to get used to hearing aids themselves, but you may have to get used to a new pattern of sounds. For some people with long-standing hearing loss, the process of reeducating the brain can be fostered by specific training or fitting techniques. Because you haven't heard certain sounds for a long time, the signals amplified by the hearing aids may sound strident, artificial, or just downright unpleasant. This "unnatural" or "harsh" quality sound you may experience can actually improve speech comprehension in the long-run, but only if you can get used to it. What hearing aids may be doing is amplifying high frequency speech sounds (like /s/, /sh/, /f/), elements of which you may not have heard, or heard differently, for years. Your hearing health care provider has a good idea of what the final amplification target should be; he or she just can't get there sometimes in one fell swoop. So, don't get discouraged if you're being asked to come back for tune-ups. Each time you return, your provider may perk up the high frequencies a little more, drop the low frequencies, or do something else to help ease your adjustment into a new auditory experience. While just actively listening to people may be enough to get you used to these new hearing sensations, you may find it helpful to engage in the kinds of "listening" practice procedures that will be discussed later. At this point, we'll discuss how you can use visual cues to improve your comprehension of speech.

Speechreading

Until recently, the preferred term for speechreading was lip-reading. We now use speechreading to emphasize the fact that when people talk, a great deal of nonverbal but important information is conveyed via facial and hand gestures, body stance, the intonation and rhythm of sentences, and the nature of the vocal emphasis placed on words and syllables. For example, the phrase "<u>where</u> are you going?" conveys quite a different meaning than "where are <u>you</u> going?" And "CONvict" has quite a different meaning than "conVICT," even though the two phrases and words look alike on the lips. Lip movements alone are insufficient to clarify the different meanings in these instances. What speechreading is, then, is lip-reading "plus." Our goal is not only to understand more of what a person is saying by looking at the lips, but also to be attuned to these other important sources of information. While much of this "tuning" may be unconscious, it is, nevertheless, very real.

If you can see a person's lips and you know the language, you have already been speechreading—to some extent. When I ask hard of hearing people if they can speechread, most deny that they are able to do it. I then proceed to show them differently. What I do is tell them that I'm going to say a month of the year. If someone gets the word wrong, I'll use a day of the week. If there is anyone who still doesn't get it (and my lips can be seen clearly—this is very important to check), I'll ask this person to tell me whether I said the numbers "three" or "four." Nobody misses this. My point is to convince you that speechreading is not some esoteric skill that one must go to school to learn. Chances are you have already been speechreading to some extent. But you can do better if you know the general principles of speechreading, and then practice them, formally or informally. But first let's talk about the general principles in speechreading. Once you're aware of these, you'll be able to appreciate their applicability in various specific situations.

Speechreading Principles

Visibility

The first general principle is that you must be able to see the lips of the person talking. Now this not only sounds simplistic, but positively insulting! Of course one has to see the lips of a person in order to speechread. But you would be surprised how many people with hearing loss, who need and can benefit from the information conveyed by lip movements, do not observe the lips of their conversational partners. They may look them "right in the eye" or simply stare off to one side. The lip movements we're trying to pick up are minuscule, rapid, and very fleeting. Because our vision is most acute at the point of focus, our best chance of perceiving these cues is by looking right at the lips. And because facial expressions, hand gestures, body stance, and so forth are larger movements, our peripheral vision should be sufficient to detect these. Try it. Look at someone's lips and note that you can also see the expression on his or her face as well as any hand movements.

Think about the implications of this simple rule. You will not be able to speechread when:
- in the dark
- a person's back is turned
- you're far from a person
- your visual acuity is poor (so, pay as much attention to your vision as to your hearing)
- a person's mouth is covered
- your conversational partner wears a full mustache and beard
- the light is in your eyes
- the head of the person you're talking to is shadowed

Any situation, in other words, which reduces the visibility of the lips is going to interfere with speechreading. How often have you, or people you know, made an extra effort, perhaps unconsciously, to ensure that you can see the person who's talking? If you have, you've been speechreading, even though you may not have known it.

Restricting Lip Movements

Anything which interferes with the movements of the lips is also going to interfere with speechreading. Some people cannot talk unless they have a pencil or the frame of eyeglasses jutting out of their mouth. Other people talk like they were practicing to be ventriloquists—their lips hardly move at all. And some people seem to talk with a perpetual smile, making speechreading almost impossible because of the way the smile distorts lip movements. In a few of these instances, a little assertiveness may help, such as, "Please take the pencil out of your mouth." But for others, it's a losing proposition—although I've often been tempted, I have not yet said, "Wipe that smile off your face!" to someone with that perennial grin. Because of the wide variations in the size and movement of the lips while talking, there are going to be large individual variations in the *speechreadability* of someone's lips. For those people with whom you have a continuing relationship, it's worth reminding them every once in a while to use more lip movements while talking. Sometimes this works quite well. For the tight-lipped stranger, this may be a futile endeavor. It may be easier to change the world than the way some people talk. So be realistic! You can't win them all, and that's okay. It's the effort you put into it that matters.

Familiarity with the Language

You can't speechread unless you know the language. This also sounds quite fundamental, and in a way it is. If you're trying to speechread someone talking in a foreign language, of course you won't be able to understand what the person is saying. But what this brings up is the notion of predictability. Since only about 30 percent of the sounds in the English language are clearly visible on the lips, even in the best of circumstances there are lots of gaps that have to be filled in. This is not quite as imposing a task as it may appear, as long as you and the person you're talking to share a common language. English is very redundant, with many linguistic and situational cues that can help us correctly predict some words we otherwise couldn't. For example, try filling in the blanks in the following sentences:

> A. Please put the dish on the _____.
> B. He hit a home _____ in the last _____.
> C. Where are you _____?
> D. It snowed again last _____.
> E. I just heard the weather report. They are _____ a major _____ tonight.

In sentence "A," someone could be saying "floor" or "bookcase," rather than "table," but this is unlikely. Sentence "E" is an example of how a previous sentence (or sentences) can improve predictability. The words are "predicting" and "storm." Now—wasn't that easy? I think this conveys the point that having an intuitive sense of the language will foster speechreading. By having an intuitive sense of the language, I don't mean that you have to be a psychic or literary genius. No matter what language you've grown up with, you can (or could more easily, prior to the onset of your hearing loss), effortlessly understand verbal messages. Don't you often fill in the last part of people's conversations before they finish? This is the kind of predictability I mean. If you're not listening to your native language, then you may have more difficulty making these predictions, as well as more difficulty understanding speech in noise or any other difficult listening situation.

Topic Restrictions

The ability to speechread improves when you can reduce conversational possibilities, as in the example above, using months, days of the week, or one of two numbers to demonstrate that we all have some ability to speechread. When you go to the bank, a travel agency, a municipal office, shopping in a clothing store, or talk to a co-worker regarding a particular project, the topics are likely to be limited by the situation. I don't suppose you talk about certificates of deposit in the clothing store, or the weather in Italy at the bank. This is not something you necessarily do consciously. The fact that topic restrictions do enter into almost any conversation should make it easier for you to speechread, and to keep from making bad guesses—if it makes no sense at all, it probably wasn't the message! Yes, a lot of guessing does take place, and sometimes, as has happened to me, I guess wrong (with occasional embarrassment but just as often, a laugh for everybody). Still, I would rather guess and keep the conversation going than give up.

It's the Message Not the Medium

When you're engaged in a conversation, don't focus on speechreading particular sounds or words. Instead, attend to the message—the meaning of what the other person is trying to convey. If you consciously try to analyze the minuscule, rapid, and fleeting movements of the lips, you're going to be three sentences behind before you figure out the missing sounds or words, if you ever do. Many books on speechreading in our profession spend an inordinate amount of time describing how different sounds of speech are made. Speechreading successfully, however, does not require you to identify all the sounds the person is forming on his or her lips. What it means is that you're able to comprehend what the person is saying. Listen to the message (the so-called "synthetic" approach to speechreading), rather than observing how different sounds are made on the lips (the "analytic" method of speechreading). Because many of the sounds of speech are either invisible, or formed exactly the same way as other sounds of speech, even the most skilled speechreader cannot identify all of them. What they do, and what you must do, is use your knowledge of the language and your awareness of topic restrictions to fill in the gaps. By focusing on the message rather than specific movements, you'll find that subsequent sentences will clarify words and sentences you may have missed.

Hearing

One extremely crucial principle in speechreading is the necessity for you to use your residual hearing as well as you can. Now, this seems like a contradiction! If we're talking about *speechreading,* why bring up *hearing*? Well, how often are you talking to someone while you're not wearing your hearing aids? Maybe late at night or early in the morning, but at most other times you're likely to be wearing them. And why would you not wear them if you know they help you? Normally, then, when conversing with other people, you're going to depend on both speechreading and hearing. And that's fine. Because our goal is to understand speech as well as we can, we should use whatever cues are available to us to realize this goal. Speechreading does not mean that you have to cut off other sources of information.

As I mentioned earlier, it's a difficult but possible task to understand speech via speechreading alone. However, many of the sounds of English are completely invisible on the lips. For example, look in the mirror while saying the word "key." It can be said with no movement at all. This is the kind of word we need context to understand—to the teenager in the house, "No you can't have the _____ to the car!" Now while you're still in front of the mirror, lip the movement to /pan/, /ban/, and /man/. They all look alike, don't they? This is where hearing comes in. It's relatively easy to hear the difference between the /b/, /p/, and /m/ sounds. In other words, what you can't see, you can hear. This is an important principle. It turns out that there are many speech sounds which are very difficult to tell apart visually, and yet are relatively easy to distinguish through hearing (i.e., while the /t/, /d/, and /n/ sounds look identical, they can be differentiated through hearing). Conversely, other sounds which are difficult to hear (like /s/, /f/, /t/, and /th/) are easy to speechread. So what we find is that vision and audition provide complementary information. What is lacking or difficult to perceive in one modality can often be picked up in the other. Therefore, depending only on speechreading, or only on hearing, may limit your ability to communicate.

In real-life situations, there are always going to be variations on how well we can see and hear someone talking. Noise will tend to mask out many speech sounds and reduce the amount of information we get through hearing. This forces us to depend more on visual cues in order to understand a spoken message. But because the loudness and type of noise is continually changing, these changes will cause your ability to understand speech to vary. In some situations you may have to rely almost entirely on vision to understand speech, while in other situations, you may be able to understand even without looking at the speaker. In other words, you have to be prepared for an unpredictable amount of hearing information due to varying noise backgrounds, as well as unpredictable visual cues. By using both vision and audition as much as possible, and any other sources of information, *most* hard of hearing people can comprehend *most* of what *most* people say in *most* situations. I'm qualifying because there will inevitably be times when you miss part or almost all of a conversation. *This will happen.* What I'm suggesting is that you think positively. Think of the occasions you can understand rather than the times you can't. That is, the glass is half full, not half empty!

Practice Procedures

There have been hundreds of books and articles purporting to teach someone how to speechread, usually extolling some unproved theory and lots of practice material. Personally, I find the practice material more convincing than the theories. Like improving or developing any skill, however, practice helps. I personally had a demonstration of the benefits of speechreading practice several months ago. For about a month I could not use my hearing aids because of a condition in both of my ear canals. All I could depend upon was speechreading (with an 85-95 dB loss in both ears, without hearing aids I'm functionally deaf). Ordinarily, I'm just a so-so speechreader. After several weeks of trying to communicate without hearing, mainly with my wife, I found my ability to speechread her noticeably improving. I still couldn't carry on an extended conversation by just speechreading, but at least in context I was able to carry on abbreviated conversations. We did cheat once in awhile and use finger spelling to clarify difficult words.

So it's very possible that speechreading practice, with and without sound, wherever and with whomever you do it, is going to help. In addition to the informal practice you get everyday when you talk to people, formal training sessions can also help. They ensure polishing of this skill and can help build your personal self-confidence by demonstrating that you *can* speechread.

I also like a procedure that is practiced "live," with a communication partner. This exercise has been termed *tracking procedures* by audiologists. Don't be turned off by the professional jargon. These are basically exercises that require you to comprehend segments of speech before proceeding to subsequent segments. In other words, you're required to "track" through a conversation in a sequential manner. The tracking exercises can be structured so that they incorporate both speechreading and communication repair strategies. Let me explain how this works.

You are sitting across from your conversational partner. The room is well lit and you're relaxed. It's going to be fun. This person has selected a paragraph as practice material; it can be from the newspaper, from a magazine article or book, or specific material related to one's vocation or interests. Whatever material is selected, it's important that the sentences follow each other in some kind of logical sequence. You should be informed of the general content or topic of the paragraph, as would be the case in real life. Now, while using a very soft voice and normal, not exaggerated lip movements (adding noise is a good idea if you can still hear the sentences), your partner should read you the first sentence of the paragraph. Did you get it all? Did you get any of it? Your job is to repeat whatever you understood of the sentence. Guess when you're not sure. You've probably made some errors but also got some words correct in the sentence.

If you missed any part of the sentence, the first step is for your partner to repeat the whole sentence again, verbatim. You may or may not get it all this time. If not, what your partner has to do is emphasize the parts you missed, increasing the duration, exaggerating the pronunciation, and so forth. For example, "Did you remember to shut off the WATER when you left the house?" Your partner keeps doing this until you get the entire sentence correct. At the beginning of the paragraph, to get the process going, you may need a few more cues. If you repeatedly miss a part of the sentence, despite the extra emphasis, your partner should give you extra hints. For example, "The word begins with a /s/ sound," or, "It's the name of a country in Europe." Paraphrasing the sentence before going back to the original version also can help.

The point is for you to be able to repeat the sentence correctly, using whatever clues necessary, including raised voice or writing the words down as last resorts. Then your partner should read the first sentence again softly, even though you now know it, but this time followed by the second sentence, the one you don't yet know. The more sentences you comprehend in a paragraph, the more the internal linguistic cues will help you understand subsequent sentences. The more practice you get, the quicker you'll be going through the process. This is a wonderful exercise for teaching concentration and identifying particular sounds and words that give you the most problems. Enjoy this process. Make it fun!

Practicing "Communication Repair" Strategies

The term "repair strategies" implies that something has broken down and has to be "repaired." What has broken down, of course, is the communication exchange. You didn't quite get all of the intended message. When you don't understand, the person you're talking to doesn't know what went wrong, or what he or she can do to correct the situation. But you should know what aspect of a person's speech made it difficult for you to understand, and you can help your conversational partner communicate more effectively with you. You can use the tracking procedure as practice in analyzing what caused the breakdowns and how they can be "repaired." Unlike the previous exercise, where your partner made modifications to try to get you to understand, in this one you have to tell your partner how his or her speech should be modified.

The rationale is simple. In real life conversation, asking "what?" or "huh?" when you don't understand doesn't often help very much. Mostly what people will do when they hear these expressions is to simply say the whole thing over and over again, maybe just as softly, quickly, or poorly articulated. In this exercise, your task is to try to figure out why you missed what you did, and then to ask your partner to make specific modifications in his or her speech. Maybe you don't need the entire sentence repeated; maybe all you didn't get was the last word. So you ask the person to repeat only the portion you missed. Or maybe your partner looked down while talking, or slurred a particular word. With a creative collaborator, you can simulate many real-life situations. Your goal is to practice "communication repair" strategies enough so that you can utilize them in everyday life. Like asking a reservations clerk in an airport to look at you when talking, or for her to talk a little louder, slower, and so forth. When you help the person you're talking to be a more effective communicator with you, you're applying the three themes I spoke about earlier, you're acknowledging your hearing loss, being assertive about your communication needs, and placing equal responsibility for the communication exchange on the person with whom you're talking.

192

Listening Practice (Auditory Training)

If we've learned anything in audiology in the past 50 years, it's that the hard of hearing person's perception of speech is not immutable. This has been dramatically illustrated to us in recent years by deaf people who have received cochlear implants. People initially report some strange auditory sensations that they're unable to identify or use. After a while, however, learning takes place. The brain "links up" to the acoustic environment and strange sounds become identifiable. While new users of hearing aids do not initially experience this dramatic shift, improvements in speech perception do take place, sometimes quite rapidly and sometimes slowly. Focused listening practice can help accelerate this process as well as stimulate the most use of a person's residual hearing.

Procedures

With a Partner

Adaptations of the previously described tracking procedure can be helpful "auditory training" procedures. In the auditory version, your partner reads you the material for you to repeat while his or her lips are covered (no visual cues). For most people, this is still going to be too easy. All right, think about situations in which you have the most difficulty understanding the spoken word—in noise, right? Okay, then that's how you should structure the tracking procedures. Perhaps the best kind of "noise" to use is narration on audio cassettes, such as books on tape. This will make the listening task difficult, as it should be. Use these recordings as background sounds and not as training stimuli. In a later section, you'll see how the same recordings can be used for self-administered auditory training.

When you miss part or all of the sentence, have your partner, a) repeat it verbatim; b) say the sentence again, this time stressing the words you missed; c) if you still miss it, the sentence should be rephrased to give you an additional cue, but then your partner should go back to the original version for you to repeat; and finally, d) let you see and hear the sentence. After you get it, your partner then starts at the beginning of the paragraph and continues the process. How long should you do this? As long as you and your partner feel comfortable. I suggest no more than 15-30 minutes in the beginning. As you well know, trying to listen under adverse circumstances can be very fatiguing.

If you have a great deal of difficulty understanding in noise, and using just your hearing is just too difficult, you may want to first try the tracking procedures when you can both see and hear your partner. Go through the same tracking process, but this time you can advise your partner to talk a little louder or slower, to repeat a certain word, to paraphrase the sentence, or to generally articulate all the syllables more precisely—anything that will help you understand. In other words, at this point you become the manager of the practice session. You'll find that as you start going through a paragraph, subsequent sentences will be easier for you to understand.

Self-Administered Auditory Training

Getting and keeping a cooperative partner can be a challenge. After awhile, you may run out of cooperative partners! Remember, though, the purpose of the training procedure is not to endanger relationships, but to foster good listening habits. You can work toward the same goal working by yourself, using available audiocassette material that comes with a written script. Years ago I used this technique to help convince severely hearing impaired children and their parents that they could use, benefit from, and develop their use of residual hearing. While we recorded our own material and wrote our own scripts, this is no longer necessary. There's lots of this kind of material out there now, for example, books on tape (unabridged) and audiotapes developed for second language learners that include a word-for-word written transcript. Check with your local bookstore or a reference librarian. You'll find that there are recorded poems, short stories, formal lectures, and so on that include verbatim written transcripts. You could apply this technique, or variation on this theme, in a few ways:

1) Most easily, all you do is listen to the tape while reading the script. This will get you used to hearing aid amplified sounds, and you may even enjoy the recording. But this doesn't present you with too much of an auditory challenge.

2) A more difficult procedure would be for you to listen to a short paragraph at a time and then read the script. What did you miss just by listening? Even though you may have missed some words, did the meaning come through? With some English as a Second Language (ESL) tapes, you're required to answer written questions to determine if you got the basic point. In addition to answering these questions, you can also check to see if you could comprehend all the words. Try to analyze the words you consistently missed; did they incorporate

specific sound elements (like some high frequency consonants) of which you should be aware?

3) An even more challenging method is to make two copies of the same script, one for you and one for your partner. Ask someone (your partner, a knowledgeable audiologist, a literate friend) to randomly white-out several words in each sentence, starting with just one word in the first sentence, then increasing the number of words eliminated in later sentences. Some of the words should be predictable from the context; others, like proper nouns, much less so. Stress the fact that you want both "easy to hear" and "hard to hear" words which have been removed with white-out. Your task is to listen to this edited script and fill in the omitted words. After you listen to the entire page, you then check the original copy to determine how well you did. This process will help you "reeducate" your hearing as you become a more focused listener.

Carry-over

What all the training procedures previously described (and not just in this section) are designed to do is to prepare you to use these techniques in real life. If your training partner is someone you talk with all the time, these suggestions can eventually carry over and make reminders unnecessary. There's some good research to indicate that this extra effort on the part of the person talking does improve speech comprehension for hard of hearing people. But even when conversing with strangers, or an infrequent communication partner, this person also wants you to understand what he or she is saying. You can be assertive in such situations without being aggressive. Put the burden on yourself. Say to them, for example, "Could you talk a little slower please. I have a hearing loss and it would make it easier for me to understand you."

This is why *it's so necessary to acknowledge your hearing loss.* You can't employ these communication strategies effectively unless you do. Don't bluff and pretend you understand. You can damage a relationship, misunderstand important instructions, and get into a heap of trouble. When it comes to important instructions, dates, names, and so forth, *even if you think you understand,* make sure you clarify just to be certain, by repeating what you think you heard. "Did you say two blue pills every three hours and three white pills every two hours?" It can make a difference!

Hearing Tactics

Hearing tactics is a term used to describe environmental manipulations that make it easier for you to understand other people. I don't mean being sneaky or manipulative in the usual sense of the word. You're reading this book because you're having difficulty in many situations and you want to do something about it. While the procedures described earlier will help, they are not the only steps you can take to help yourself. Most likely, as you interact with other people in a number of situations, you're still going to have some difficulty hearing everything that's going on. Like military tactics, using hearing tactics means that you plan ahead, marshal your resources, and engage the "enemy"—the difficult communication situation. Now, no hearing tactic, or any hearing device for that matter, will eliminate all of your hearing problems. But you can take a giant step toward reducing many of them by understanding how you can exert more control over the communicative situation. Here are some examples:

Move closer

Always try to get closer to the person talking, but do respect their "personal space!" This is an underestimated but valuable technique. For example, in the average room, if you're eight feet from someone speaking and you can move to within four feet of this person, you've increased the sound pressure at the microphone of your hearing aids by 6 dB. If you can get within two feet of the speaker, then the increase is 12 dB—a rather significant boost. I really don't recommend getting much closer unless you have a "special relationship" to this individual! While it's true that some modern hearing aids will compensate for distance by increasing amplification of weaker sounds, and decreasing the amplification of stronger sounds, they will also amplify strong and weak background noises in a similar fashion. Better comprehension results when the sound you want to hear is located close to the hearing aid microphone, whether this sound is a person talking, a television set, radio, or anything else.

Quiet the Room

This is a principle that applies just about every place you go. When you walk into a restaurant for a relaxing meal and you find that the young staff is playing their favorite loud music through the P.A. system, what do you do? Here's where assertiveness pays off. Many young people seem completely unaware that there *is* loud music in the background—this all seems very normal to them. When it's explained that the music makes speech comprehension virtually impossible for the person with a hearing loss, more often than not they graciously comply with the request. Hopefully, after a few such requests, they may learn to appreciate the "sounds of silence." Wouldn't it be nice to have "noise-free" areas in the same way we now have "smoke-free" restaurants? When you arrive, look or ask for the quietest table. The hostess usually knows. Don't sit in the middle of a room with parties all around you. Stay away from any extra noise-producing areas such as the kitchen, background piano music, an air conditioner or heating system. Better yet, look for places to eat that encourage private conversations; restaurants do differ in their sensitivity to noise. Seat yourself in the center of your group where it's easy for you to see and hear everyone.

Many people feel that they have to have the stereo turned on when entertaining people in their home. A gentle reminder to turn it off usually suffices. In a family gathering, the youngsters may have the television set turned up while ignoring it; if it's your house, pull the plug and/or move the youngsters to another room. If it's not your house, you have to be a little more diplomatic; either the television set should be turned down or off, or try to move your personal conversation to a quieter area in the house. Whatever house you happen to be in, make sure you have a good sight-line to all the guests. Don't sit at the end of a long couch, you won't be able to see or hear the person at the other end. If only a small group is involved, try to get some conversational "rules" established. If these people are friends, you can ask that only one person at a time talk. "Cross-conversation" presents, perhaps, the most difficult situation for people with hearing loss.

Senior centers and retirement homes, particularly those that serve meals, often present a challenging communication environment. In such places, the acoustical conditions can be improved by: a) acoustical treatment on ceilings and walls; b) rugs, if possible, on the floor; c) if not possible, then rubber coasters on chair and table legs; d) placing a felt, or some other soft map, on dining tables under the tablecloths which will reduce the clattering sounds of dishes and silverware; and e) sitting at a smaller (4-person) rather than larger table (8-person) during dining activities.

Advance Planning

Do some anticipatory planning for any activity. For example, before you attend any large area listening situation (theater, lecture, house of worship, etc.) call ahead to see if they have an assistive listening device available. What these devices do is basically transmit the sound to a special radio or infrared receiver that you're wearing, reducing the loss of acoustical clarity which occurs when the sound emanates from a loudspeaker some distance from you. In most such places, by law according to the American's with Disabilities Act (ADA), they're required to have such devices available. However, houses of worship are an exception, yet many make such devices available as a moral obligation. I personally would not attend any large area listening situation without ensuring that such devices were available. Without one, I either don't know what's going on or I'm straining so hard to hear that I don't enjoy the activity or performance.

Microphone Technique

Even though an assistive listening device is available in an auditorium, and the signal is being transmitted to a special radio or infrared receiver, this doesn't always take care of the problems that may occur. It will if the sound is coming from a movie soundtrack or other recorded material. But if the source is a person using a microphone, you may have an additional problem, one that will fully challenge your willingness to be reasonably assertive about your communication needs. What I'm referring to is the abysmal lack of proper microphone technique, even by people who should know better. In any large area listening situation, the lack of good microphone technique is often the weakest link in the communication chain. What seems to happen is that talkers get so wrapped up in what they're saying, they forget that there's a microphone on the podium. Most of these are low-sensitivity microphones, requiring a talker to be within four to six inches of it for effective pick-up. Or if it's a hand-held microphone, many people wave it around as if it were a baton or a pointer—everywhere but close to their mouth. So what do you do?

- You arrive a little earlier and remind the event organizer, the speaker, or the minister, of the necessity for the person talking to stay close to the microphone while talking.
- During the talk, they're going to forget themselves and walk away from the microphone while still speaking. You ask loudly but politely for the speaker to get closer to the microphone. Other people in the audience will appreciate your assertiveness because of their own difficulty hearing.
- If a lapel instead of a podium microphone is available, ask that it be used and pinned close to the person's mouth.

- If there's a public question and answer period after the talk and you can't hear the questions, don't suffer in silence. Ask, again politely, that the questions be repeated before the answer is given. Remember, you're probably not the only one in the audience who can't hear the questions.

In the last hearing aid orientation group which I held, I was given an excellent example of poor microphone technique and how a bit of assertiveness serves everyone's purpose. One of the participants complained that he never heard the homilies prepared by the same two women in his church. Their voices were soft and they typically sat two feet or so away from the microphone. Every Sunday, he said, he just sat there and waited for them to finish, not understanding a word. His normal hearing wife then piped up and said, "I never understand them either and I don't think anyone else can!" Before the next service, the husband asked the two women to talk right into the microphone as he was having difficulty understanding them. That Sunday, not only my patient, but everyone heard the women loud and clear.

Wrap up

In this church anecdote, we have an example of the three themes with which I began this chapter. The hard of hearing person had to acknowledge the hearing loss, had to be assertive in approaching women, and all effort served the purposes of both parties in the communication exchange. The lesson in this example is that you, as a hard of hearing person, have to be more than a passive recipient of "services." You have to take more control over your own listening needs. Work closely with your hearing health care professionals. They have information and skills that will help you.

No—magic wands are not available to "wave" away your hearing loss, but with the appropriate use of modern technology and the judicious use of appropriate communication strategies, you can go a long way in reducing the impact hearing loss is having in your life.

CHAPTER ELEVEN
Tinnitus

Richard S. Tyler, Ph.D.

Dr. Tyler earned undergraduate and graduate degrees in Communication Disorders and Audiology at the University of Western Ontario, and his Doctorate in Psychoacoustics at the University of Iowa. He's currently Professor and Director of Audiology in the Department of Otolaryngology--Head & Neck Surgery at the University of Iowa, and Professor in the Department of Speech Pathology and Audiology. Dr. Tyler has authored over 160 articles and has been author/editor of books on assistive devices for the hearing impaired and cochlear implants. He's been a visiting scholar in countries around the world. Presently, he's restoring the Secrest 1883 Octagonal Barn, one of the oldest and largest octagonal barns in the United States.

Profile of the Tinnitus Sufferer

People and their tinnitus come in all shapes and sizes. Some hear soft, high-pitched whistles while others hear combinations of sounds that include bacon frying, horns and crickets all in one. The most remarkable dimension on which people differ is the degree to which they're bothered by their tinnitus. For some, it rests gently in the back of their mind, whereas others cannot concentrate sufficiently to hold down a job. Table 11-I shows some of the most common problems reported by tinnitus patients. The most often reported problem is difficulty falling asleep. Patients also have difficulty concentrating and are agitated by the noise in their head. It's noteworthy that some patients complain about being in a quiet place whereas others complain about being in a noisy place. The three main effects, being tired, not being able to concentrate, and being annoyed by their tinnitus, can play havoc with one's life.

Nearly all people with tinnitus have hearing loss. Frustration with not hearing well, and the stress created by having to strain in order to listen carefully, further complicate the plight of the tinnitus sufferer. In addition, many people with tinnitus find that loud sounds are heard as being very loud, sometimes painful. This is called *hyperacusis*. It can cause people to fear loud sounds or to avoid places they might experience loud noises.

There are many secondary effects of tinnitus. These include problems functioning at work; difficulty communicating; alcohol and drug abuse; and problems in personal relationships. Sometimes the question is posed, "Which came first, the tinnitus or the psychological problems?" Tinnitus results from a real disease and, I believe, in most situations the tinnitus came first. Obviously, some people who have psychological problems will get tinnitus, and there are many people with psychological problems who do not have tinnitus. Psychological problems are probably better viewed on a continuum, which of us is free of psychological and emotional stresses, and would not hope to learn better ways of coping?

Table 11-I.

Common Problems reported by tinnitus patients. There were 72 patients sampled in the study (Tyler and Baker, 1983).

Problem	Percent of Patients
Getting to Sleep	56.9
Persistence of Tinnitus	48.6
Understanding Speech	37.5
Despair, Frustration, Depression	36.1
Annoyance, Irritation, Inability to Relax	34.7
Concentration, Confusion	33.3
Dependence on Drugs	23.6
Pain/Headaches	18.0
Worse upon Awakening in Morning	16.6
Insecurity, Fear, Worry	16.6
Avoid Noisy Situations	15.3
Withdraw, Avoid Friends	13.8
Understanding Television	11.1
Avoid Quiet Situations	11.1

Prevalence

Tinnitus is very common in the general population. About 15 to 20 percent (almost 1 person in every 5) report hearing more than a temporary tinnitus. About 5 percent (1 person in every 20) report tinnitus with severe annoyance, and about 0.5 percent (1 person in about 200) report a tinnitus that has a severe effect on their lives. Actually, the prevalence is much higher in people over the age of 55 years. Over 40 percent (about 1 person in every 3) of this age group report tinnitus. In general, older hearing impaired people with a history of noise exposure are most likely to have tinnitus.

Classification

Some classifications of tinnitus use *subjective* and *objective* terminology. Subjective tinnitus can only be heard by the person with it, whereas objective tinnitus can be heard by someone listening with a stethoscope or microphone at the external ear canal. I don't think this is a useful distinction. As you noted in Chapter Four by Dr. Mueller, the ear is divided into three parts: the outer ear, the middle ear, and the inner. The hearing nerve then connects the inner ear to nerve fibers which go to the brain. I prefer to classify tinnitus in a way similar to which we classify hearing loss. We can have a middle ear tinnitus, a sensorineural tinnitus or a central tinnitus. Middle ear tinnitus has its origins in the air-filled cavity behind the eardrum. Two examples of this are sounds that are produced by abnormal muscle twitching or abnormal blood flow. Sensorineural tinnitus has its origins in the sensory or neural system. The sensory organ of hearing is the inner ear, the snail-shaped cochlea containing hair cells and nerve endings. The neural system of hearing includes the hearing nerves that connect the inner ear to the brain. Central tinnitus has its origins in the brain.

Causes

Almost anything that causes hearing loss can cause tinnitus. Most causes of tinnitus are idiopathic, that is, they're unknown. A few of the more common causes are described below, but most are difficult to specify exactly, or are unknown.

Noise

The most common cause is noise exposure. Working in an excessively noisy environment, such as a factory, for many years, can cause a progressive hearing loss, often accompanied by tinnitus. The onset of tinnitus can precede the presence of hearing loss, or tinnitus can begin long after the hearing loss. Many recreational hobbies can cause tinnitus, such as snowmobiles, lawn mowers, and chain saws, as well as musicians playing in orchestras or rock bands. Audiences attending loud concerts can also be at risk for noise-induced tinnitus, particularly if their seats are near loudspeakers or in regions of the auditorium, such as in some corners, where sound levels can be enhanced. People who use guns, either in their vocation (e.g. the military or law enforcement) are particularly at risk. Finally, it should be noted that even a single exposure to a loud burst of noise can result in hearing loss and tinnitus. I've seen a patient who was under a sink fixing the plumbing when someone turned on a loud trash compactor. Permanent tinnitus resulted.

Sometimes there's a temporary "ringing" in the ears during or following exposure to loud sound. This should be considered a warning, and you should immediately vacate such an environment and not return without hearing protection.

Noise-induced tinnitus can often be prevented. In the next chapter, Dr. Campbell nicely addresses hearing protectors and their noise ratings. Read the labels and buy the ones that produce lower noise levels. And wear hearing protection whenever you're around loud noise. The fact that you don't experience pain or discomfort should not mislead you into believing you are safe. Hearing loss in higher frequencies is often a painless experience, and a most common result is tinnitus. Furthermore, these devastating effects on the inner ear hair cells are accumulative. After several years, it doesn't take much to add up to tinnitus or impaired hearing. Take precaution before it's too late.

Medications

Other causes include some medications. There are a few medications that are considered ototoxic, that is, they're known to impair hearing. These are usually prescribed only when they're absolutely necessary. Other prescribed medications may carry an uncommon side effect of hearing loss and tinnitus. You should ask the physician prescribing any medications about these possibilities, and when taking new medications, be alert for the onset or worsening of your hearing or tinnitus.

Some over-the-counter medications can exacerbate tinnitus. Aspirin is a common example of this, but there are others. Read labels carefully. If symptoms develop, discuss these changes immediately with your physician. Also, for details on potential ototoxic drugs, I encourage you to read the next chapter.

Temporomandibular Joint [TMJ] Dysfunction

There have been dentists who argue that some patients have a dysfunction of the joint connecting their jaw to the bone under the ear—the temporomandibular joint. Tinnitus can arise, they purport, even when the joint is motionless. However, the mechanism by which this might cause tinnitus is obscure. There is no evidence to suggest that an abnormality of the TMJ causes tinnitus or that any form of treatment of this joint cures or reduces tinnitus. Nevertheless, some patients report relief from TMJ treatment. Healthy skepticism is advised at this point. Controlled studies and a physiological explanation are needed.

Other Causes

There are many causes of tinnitus other than noise exposure and medications. The normal aging process, presbycusis, can result in tinnitus as well as hearing loss. Other causes include Meniere's Disease (hearing loss, balance disorder and tinnitus), perilymph fistula (a hole in the inner ear allowing fluid to escape) and head trauma.

How Tinnitus is Measured

Many people without tinnitus at first think that maybe the sound is imagined. Maybe it's "psychological," or just made up. This is not so. Tinnitus can be measured and quantified. This is often reassuring to people with tinnitus, and helps partners, family and friends appreciate that tinnitus is real.

Pitch, Loudness and Quality

Because tinnitus is a sound, it shares attributes with other sounds, including pitch, loudness, and quality. Even though tinnitus may be composed of many sounds, on tone-generating equipment, it's possible to adjust the frequency of a pure tone to match the same pitch as the most prominent pitch of the tinnitus. Similarly, it's possible to adjust the level of a pure tone so that it has the same loudness as the tinnitus. This quantification of tinnitus can be useful to monitor changes over time.

In most patients, tinnitus can also be masked. That is, it's possible to present an external noise so that it covers up or "masks" the tinnitus. For some people, this is quite a breathtaking experience because it's the first time they have not heard the tinnitus in years. Unfortunately, in almost all cases, the tinnitus returns when the noise is turned off. You should be warned that playing loud noise can also make your tinnitus worse, so do not try this on your own. This should be done under the direction of a clinical audiologist trained in tinnitus treatment.

Otoacoustic Emissions

In recent years, it has been discovered that the cochlea can emit a sound which is transmitted backwards through the middle ear and into the external ear canal. This spontaneous otoacoustic emission, as it's called, is apparently a sign of a normal healthy ear. It is typically very soft, less than 5 or 10 dB (HL) when measured in the ear canal. Even a mild hearing loss often eliminates the emission. Most people with tinnitus also have a hearing loss, and therefore generally do not have an otoacoustic emission. However, there are a few people, maybe less than one percent of tinnitus sufferers, who have a tinnitus directly related to their spontaneous otoacoustic emission. There have been reports of some humans and some animals who have very loud otoacoustic emissions that can be heard by others in the same room!

How is Tinnitus Represented in the Auditory System?

Actually, no one knows for sure how tinnitus is represented or coded in the hearing nerve or brain. Information is normally sent from the inner ear (the cochlea) to the brain by brief electrical impulses. In the absence of sound, there are some low-level spontaneous impulses sent from the inner ear to the brain. These are infrequent, and the brain has learned to ignore this spontaneous activity. These spontaneous impulses are normally not "heard." When a sound is presented, many impulses are created in the inner ear and sent to the brain. Once there, the brain "tells" you that a sound has been presented.

One theory about the coding of tinnitus is that the spontaneous activity of these impulses on the hearing nerve is at an abnormally high level, even without any sound. The brain interprets this activity as sound, or tinnitus. Actually, the abnormal spontaneous activity might even originate in the brain itself. Figure 11-1 shows an example of nerve fiber impulses that might relate to tinnitus.

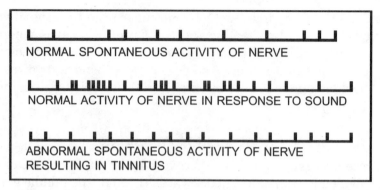

NORMAL SPONTANEOUS ACTIVITY OF NERVE

NORMAL ACTIVITY OF NERVE IN RESPONSE TO SOUND

ABNORMAL SPONTANEOUS ACTIVITY OF NERVE
RESULTING IN TINNITUS

Figure 11-1: Hypothetical nerve fiber activity, shown as spikes as a function of time.

Medical Treatments

Medications

There is no medication that has been shown to be an effective treatment for tinnitus. To qualify as an effective treatment, a medication has to be compared to a control or placebo. Although many newspaper reports routinely claim a cure has been discovered for tinnitus, these medications are later found to be no more effective than a sugar pill. Scientific studies are essential. We need to remind ourselves that tinnitus is a symptom. It is likely caused by many different things and may have many different physiological mechanisms involved. Therefore, no single medication is likely to work for everyone.

Some patients and otolaryngologists report that certain medications work for some patients. It's important to determine if this is true or not. Under the supervision of your physician, you could try a particular drug, and after a few weeks, if you observe benefit, stop taking it to see if the tinnitus returns. If it does, it could indicate some value in what you were taking. Medication can be used effectively to help people cope with tinnitus, even though the tinnitus itself might not change.

Tinnitus causes all kinds of problems in people's lives, including difficulty getting to sleep, depression and anxiety. There are a variety of medications that can help in these areas. It's important to be treated by a physician, preferably an ear-nose and throat specialist. If you plan to use drug therapy, ask your physician what the medication is and its potential side effects. Important research continues on the effectiveness of different medications, and we can hope that some day a cure will be found.

Surgery

There are a few causes of tinnitus that can be treated surgically. These causes might involve muscle twitching, blood vessel abnormalities, or nerve tumors. The middle ear contains muscles that can spontaneously twitch. If this is the cause, these muscles can be cut which should eliminate the tinnitus. However, the middle ear muscles normally offer some protection from very loud, abrupt sounds, and this protection will be reduced by such surgical intervention. This should be considered when weighing the potential benefits of this procedure.

On occasion, abnormal blood flow in the middle ear is audible. Sometimes, there's an abnormal new growth behind the eardrum (such as a vascular neoplasm), or the development of a proliferation of blood vessels (arteriovenous malformations), or the perception of the flow of blood through vessels (venous hum). It is sometimes possible to surgically intervene and correct this. Some people find their tinnitus so severe and distressing that they're prepared to eliminate their hearing in the affected ear with the hope of attaining relief. In this case, a surgeon cuts the hearing nerve, resulting in a total loss of hearing for that ear. Most unfortunately, in more than 50 percent of these cases, the tinnitus persists.

Electrical Stimulation

Research studies have clearly shown that electrical activity presented near the cochlea can reduce tinnitus. Although the precise mechanism of this is elusive, the normal cochlea contains several electrical potentials which could be altered. Experimental trials have included electrode placement on the eardrum and through a hole in the eardrum to allow placement on the interior wall of the middle ear cavity near the cochlea. Cochlear implants (artificial hearing for those who are deaf and who are largely unable to benefit from hearing aids), have also been shown to reduce tinnitus in some patients. A few wearable devices for electrical suppression of tinnitus have been developed. Although not commercially available at this time, it's hoped that they will be in the near future.

Acupuncture

Acupuncture has been shown to be effective in reducing pain, and it was therefore reasonable to hope that it might also reduce tinnitus. However, several controlled investigations have shown that acupuncture is not effective for the treatment of tinnitus or sensorineural hearing loss.

Non-Medical Approaches to Tinnitus Relief

Hearing Aids

As mentioned earlier, most people with tinnitus also have a hearing loss and will therefore benefit from hearing aids. Amplification will improve communication, which has two important indirect effects: being able to communicate more easily, and not having to strain to listen closely which often reduces stress. In addition, hearing aids produce small amounts of background noise, and also amplify background environmental sounds. This acoustic ambience can facilitate therapy based on decreasing the tinnitus loudness, or distraction, or masking.

Masking

Early in the search for treatment, patients were reporting that listening to music, traffic noise and conversation distracted them from their tinnitus. This in itself is now a recommended treatment. It's something you can easily do—and may be already doing. Find out which background sounds help you. They can be tape-recorded to capture the specific sound that works for you. Or it may simply be easier to buy pre-recorded audiotapes of such sounds as waves rolling up on the beach, rain pouring down on leaves, or other pleasant sounds. If the sound disturbs others, you can use a portable compact tape player with earphones where it can be played in your kitchen, living room, bedroom or office.

Because some patients have reported that their tinnitus was less disturbing in the presence of background noise, a behind-the-ear hearing aid-like device was developed which produces noise. In such cases, like music in a room, the external noise through the masker device (worn like a hearing aid) covered up the internal sound of the tinnitus. Later models were developed for in-the-ear fittings like ITE hearing aids.

It's speculated that masking probably works by activating the nerve fibers that would otherwise convey the tinnitus information. In some cases, only "partial" masking works, where the tinnitus is still present, but reduced in loudness. In lieu of the tinnitus, the masking noise is audible. Thus, those who suffer from tinnitus must decide which noise they prefer, the tinnitus or the masking. The masker usually is a wide frequency range sound like a fan, whereas the tinnitus may sound like a screeching noise. Each person must decide for themselves if they are a candidate for masking. In masking therapy, once the masker is removed, the tinnitus typically returns to its previous level (although sometimes after a few hours of relief). In a few patients, when the masker is turned off, the tinnitus can be worse, and this sometimes prevents patients from seeking the benefits of this treatment.

Biofeedback

Biofeedback involves measuring some biological function of your body and providing you with feedback about that function. For example, when you clench your fist, the muscle tension in your arm increases. The amount of muscle tension in your arm can be measured with wires placed on its surface. The two wires simply measure the voltage (electrical activity) between the wires, which is directly related to muscle tension. The amount of electrical activity in the wires (and therefore the amount of tension in your arm) can be used to control the intensity of a light source. As you relax the muscle, the intensity of the light gets weaker. When you clench your fist tightly, the intensity of the light gets brighter.

Biofeedback has been used to help tinnitus patients learn to relax. They can be made aware of when they are tense, and which muscles are tense. They have also been shown how to relax these muscles. The biofeedback tells them when they're relaxing certain muscles, and how effective they are at relaxing. After a person knows how to relax their muscles, they no longer need to be connected to the wires. Some people may want to return for a "refresher" at later times. Although biofeedback usually does not do away with tinnitus, the ability to relax is very helpful to many patients.

Biofeedback is best done by someone experienced in biofeedback therapy, usually a clinical psychologist (and some audiologists). While some psychologists may need an explanation of tinnitus, they are effective in teaching relaxation techniques for many purposes.

Counseling and Cognitive Behavior Modification

A variety of counseling techniques are available to help tinnitus patients. These typically involve understanding the particular problems of the patient, examining the social and work environment, and setting clear and achievable goals. It can be important to distinguish between hearing the tinnitus and the patient's reaction to it. This approach accepts that the tinnitus is there and that it cannot be changed. However, *a person's reaction to their tinnitus can be changed.* Cognitive behavior modification works on techniques to help patients learn to change their reaction.

Generally, clinical psychologists are trained to provide these kinds of therapies, although some audiologists and psychiatrists may also have such experience. If the psychologist has no knowledge about tinnitus, introduce him or her to your clinical audiologist. You might also consider inviting them to a self-help group, either as a guest speaker or an observer.

Habituation Therapy

Habituation is the decrease in a response to a stimulus after repeated exposures. For example, when you begin driving a car, the traffic noise can be loud. After driving for a few minutes, the traffic noise fades into the background. Another example is when a person initially startles to the sound of a door slamming shut. After hearing the sound several times, however, they no longer startle. Habituation typically does not occur if the stimulus has some important aversive significance, such as a gun shot, or if the person is afraid of the stimulus.

Hallam, Rachman and Hinchcliffe (1984) and Carlsson and Erlandsson (1991) suggest that many patients naturally habituate to their tinnitus. Jastreboff and Hazell (1993) have proposed the use of habituation for tinnitus treatment.

There are two stages to the habituation approach. First, counseling should eliminate or reduce the fear of tinnitus. This is necessary before habituation can begin. The tinnitus can still be annoying and bothersome, but the patient shouldn't feel threatened by it or feel that it indicates something threatening or dangerous.

Second, the tinnitus patient should be continuously exposed to low levels of background noise. The tinnitus should be just audible above the noise, so that they're perceived as one sound by the brain. After several months, the patient should grow accustomed to both the noise and the tinnitus. The low-level noise can be produced by a wearable noise generator (such as the masker discussed earlier, or a stereo earphone). The noise source can also be environmentally-based (such as the static occurring between stations on a radio).

Habituation therapy differs from masking therapy in some important ways. Masking is intended to cover up the tinnitus entirely or to reduce its loudness, whichever is preferred by the patient. Masking has an immediate effect. When the masking noise is turned off, it is expected that the tinnitus returns. In habituation therapy, it's important to hear the tinnitus just above the background noise. This way the brain can habituate to the background noise and tinnitus, and learn to ignore them both. When the noise-generating device is removed after several months of therapy, the intent is for the tinnitus to be gone or reduced in loudness.

Keep Focused on Activities

We can often choose how to occupy our time. When we have nothing to do but sit and think about our problems, many of us can experience depression. If we focus on our tinnitus, how terrible it sounds, how life is unfair, and how we are stuck with it, it's easy to appreciate how sad and helpless we feel.

Conversely, when we're engaged in an activity we find interesting and enjoyable, there's less time to worry about other problems in our life. Many tinnitus patients already know this, and are very successful in pursuing pleasurable pastimes, hobbies or events. The chosen activity should be absorbing to the extent that you forget about the tinnitus, but it should not be too demanding such that it produces stress. If we're concentrating on television, pottery, reading, carpentry, sewing or conversation, there's simply less focus on tinnitus.

Reduce Stress

Too much stress in our lives can take its toll on many aspects of our health. Many tinnitus sufferers complain that their tinnitus is worse when they experience stress. Furthermore, many sufferers report that when their stress is reduced, their tinnitus is less. There are many clinics offering stress reduction therapy and many good self-help books on this stress management. Although it's not possible to avoid all stress (and likely not desirable), its management is a good thing for most tinnitus patients.

Get Plenty of Rest

One of the most common complaints from those suffering from tinnitus is that their internal noise makes it difficult for them to fall asleep. Many also report that when they're tired, their tinnitus is worse. Therefore, it's important that tinnitus patients develop strategies for getting adequate rest. Although the plan will depend on the individual, options include playing pre-recorded soft and relaxing background music or noise (as described earlier) which can be set on a timer to go off after sleep is achieved. If home remedies don't work or aren't for you, you might consider attending a sleep clinic or taking medications under medical supervision.

Examine your Food and Drinks

Many patients report that changes in their diet result in improvements in their tinnitus. Of course, it's important to maintain a healthy diet, so don't change anything that would jeopardize this. If in doubt, you should check with a professional who is knowledgeable about food, nutrition and diets.

Some patients report that when they stop drinking coffee, their tinnitus is reduced. For other patients it might be alcohol, smoking, fatty foods or something else. I ask patients to explore for themselves what they think might be helpful. For example, you might stop drinking coffee for a month. If that doesn't work, something else can be tried. Experiment with one thing at a time, and allow long enough for it to take hold. I do caution you that trying to give up alcohol or coffee, for many people, can be emotionally and physically challenging. These kinds of changes need to be under appropriate, watchful supervision, such as a professional who understands addiction.

Self-Help Groups

There is some concern that self-help groups can focus people on the problem of tinnitus, and not on helpful ways of its treatment. Unless professionals are involved, the risk of misinformation exists. Therefore, it's probably in your best interest to have a professional involved in the group, such as a clinical audiologist, psychologist, therapist or other clinician knowledgeable about tinnitus.

References

Carlsson S.G. and Erlandsson S.I. Habituation and tinnitus: an experimental study. Journal of Psychosomatic Research, Vol.35, 509-514, 1991.

Hallam, R., Rachman, S. and Hinchcliffe, R. Psychological aspects of tinnitus. In S. Rachman, *Contributions to Medical Psychology*, Oxford: Pergamon Press, 1984.

Jastreboff P.J., and Hazell, J.W.P. A neurophysiological approach to tinnitus: clinical implications. British Journal of Audiology, Vol. 27, 7-17, 1993.

Tyler, R.S. and Baker, L. J. Difficulties experienced by tinnitus sufferers. Journal of Speech and Hearing Disorders, Vol. 48, 148-154, 1983.

CHAPTER TWELVE
Preventing Hearing Loss
Kathleen C.M. Campbell, Ph.D.

Dr. Campbell is Professor and Director of Audiology at Southern Illinois University School of Medicine in Springfield. She obtained her Doctorate in Audiology and Hearing Science at the University of Iowa. In 1989, she started the Audiology program at Southern Illinois University School of Medicine. Dr. Campbell publishes extensively in the area of electrophysiologic measures, ototoxicity, and other auditory pathologies. She and her husband live a quiet life in the country outside of Springfield where they're attempting to raise their cat, Spike, to become a model citizen (but have been less successful in that endeavor).

As with most problems, "An ounce of prevention is worth a pound of cure." Although you can't always prevent hearing loss, there are many things you can do to reduce the risk. One thing is to be aware of which drugs and chemicals can affect hearing. In some cases, certain medications can increase your risk of hearing loss but may be necessary to treat your particular medical condition. Your knowledge of the possible side effect can help you be prepared for any problems that develop and may lay the foundation for more informed decisions and discussions with your physician. Your knowledge of possible side effects of over-the-counter drugs may give you insights into the quantity of drugs you currently take, and perhaps, you might recognize a problem sooner. In addition, knowing which environmental and industrial chemicals may damage hearing can help you avoid exposure or improve decisions about how often to have your hearing tested.

Another protection of hearing is limiting your exposure to loud noise. We live in an increasingly noisy world which, in many cases, is putting our hearing at risk. Yet, many of us are too shy to ask to have the volume turned down at a movie or concert or to simply leave. Worse yet, we expose ourselves to noise with chain saws, boom boxes, motorcycles, and a variety of other machines and don't wear hearing protection, although it is readily available. We've known for many years that loud noise exposure can cause permanent hearing loss (Dobie, 1993), but because it's only legally regulated in the work place, non-work exposure continues.

Part I: Preventing Drug-Induced Hearing Loss

Some of the medications we use are ototoxic, which means that they're harmful or toxic to the ear (Campbell, 1993; Campbell and Durrant, 1993). Usually when we say that a drug is ototoxic, we mean that it causes hearing loss but it can also indicate that the drug affects the vestibular (balance) portion of the ear or causes ringing in the ears (tinnitus). Some drugs cause all three symptoms while others are fairly specific causing only hearing loss and tinnitus, or only balance problems.

If you wondered why someone would be given a medication with this possible side effect, there are many reasons. Sometimes the drug can be ototoxic but the side effect is very rare. Just as in noise-induced hearing loss, there's a great deal of variability in individual susceptibility and we often don't know why. Whenever a medication is selected, the possible risk must be weighed against the hopeful benefit. If the risk of ototoxicity is low, your need for the medication may exceed the risk.

Hearing Loss Induced by Medications

Aspirin

Sometimes, medications are known to be ototoxic but only when they're used at high dosage levels. For example, it's well known that aspirin can cause hearing loss and tinnitus when given at high levels (Jung et al., 1993). Most of us never notice this side effect because we only occasionally take one or two aspirin. However, if you take many aspirin you may notice a ringing or "ocean sound" in your ears. If you continue to take a lot of aspirin, you may notice a decrease in your hearing. But most of us can take aspirin on and off for our entire lives and never experience side effects. So for us, aspirin intake is not an issue. Typically, the symptoms of hearing loss and tinnitus with excessive aspirin use will dissipate upon termination of use. Therefore, the chance of permanent hearing loss or tinnitus from aspirin is extremely unlikely.

But very low doses of aspirin may not be effective in the person with arthritis or other inflammation. Aspirin is sometimes recommended in these cases for a variety of reasons; it's inexpensive, readily available, and is often quite effective. However, it does require that you keep an eye on your dosage levels.

Chemotherapy

There are many drugs used for chemotherapy which do not cause hearing loss or do so very infrequently. Some chemotherapeutic drugs, like nitrogen mustard or DFMO, can cause hearing loss but are not in widespread use. However, chemotherapeutic drugs containing platinum compounds (for example, cisplatin and carboplatin), are commonly used and can frequently cause hearing loss. Of these drugs, the most commonly used is cisplatin. It is used in a variety of cancers including bladder cancer, various head and neck and brain cancers, some lung cancers, testicular cancer, ovarian cancer, and many other gynecological cancers. It's very ototoxic but is often the most effective, or the only effective agent in treating certain types of cancer. Because it is so effective, it has wider use in various types of cancers in adults, and even in children. Of course, the good news is that some cancers which used to be incurable can now be cured. However, the downside is that a high percentage of these patients survive with hearing loss.

The degree of risk is proportional to a number of factors. Perhaps the biggest factor is the total amount of cisplatin used. But kidney function, general health, age, pigmentation (blue-eyed or brown-eyed) and other factors may come into play. Even if you knew that you were at very high risk for hearing loss, you would probably proceed with chemotherapy, realizing it could save or prolong your life.

So, the question really is: if you know that you or your family member will be getting chemotherapy which could cause hearing loss, what can you do? Cisplatin-induced hearing loss is almost always permanent. Therefore, you need to do everything you can to prevent it. First, I would recommend not being exposed to loud noise. We know from animal studies that if you administer a dose of cisplatin that should be too low to cause hearing loss, and you administer a level and duration of noise that should be too low to impair hearing, the combination can still result in hearing loss. However, normal conversational-level speech shouldn't be loud enough to impair hearing. Also, because cisplatin can cause delayed hearing loss, and may be retained in the ears for some months after chemotherapy has stopped, I would recommend no noise exposure for at least six months after you cease chemotherapy.

As part of preventing cisplatin-induced hearing loss, hearing should be tested before, during, and after treatment. Audiologic monitoring starts with a good baseline evaluation prior to the first round of chemotherapy. It can consist of pure tones, and various speech testing, which become the reference points for subsequent changes in hearing. Especially important to measure are high frequencies since they're often involved in ototoxicity.

There are various protocols for monitoring hearing, and they may change depending on your needs and dosing schedule. After your baseline hearing is established, you'll return prior to each round of treatment. This is ideal because it's when you're feeling your best, you can concentrate on listening tests, and your hearing (which may fluctuate somewhat during chemotherapy) has had time to stablize since the last treatment. You'll also be tested again at the end of chemotherapy, and a few months down the line to check for any delayed or progressive hearing loss.

Another approach in detecting ototoxic changes is a new test technique called "otoacoustic emissions," or OAEs (discussed by Dr. Mueller in Chapter 4). By placing a tiny microphone in your ear canal, we can read and measure the sounds your ear produces. If the inner ear becomes damaged, the OAEs will diminish or disappear completely. OAEs are a wonderful test for ototoxicity for several reasons. For one thing, they *only* measure cochlear function, and the cochlea is the area of the ear most vulnerable to ototoxic drugs. Also, when ototoxic drugs are used, the OAEs have been shown to diminish or disappear before hearing loss is found.

Antibiotics

Most antibiotics very rarely impair hearing. However, one category of antibiotics known as "aminoglycosides" *can* cause hearing loss. These drugs were developed in the 1940s, and represented a big step in the war against infectious diseases, and in fact cured infections that were previously untreatable. The risk of ototoxicity really varies according to the type of aminoglycoside antibiotic used. Today, we know much more about these drugs and their associated effects on hearing than we did a few decades ago. Physicians can now make good decisions in selecting the appropriate drug most likely to cure an infection without damaging your hearing.

In general, aminoglycoside antibiotics, even when used in long-term treatment (over one week) for severe infections, have a relatively low risk of causing hearing loss. When very short-term treatment (a day or two) is administered just prior to surgery to prevent infection, the risk of damaging hearing is extremely low. Long-term treatment is usually reserved for conditions like severe bacterial pneumonia which doesn't respond to other treatments, or more commonly for osteomyelitis which is an infection of the bone. In these cases, auditory function is monitored in the same way as for chemotherapy except you're tested once or twice each week because of daily drug administration. Also, because these drugs stay in the inner ear for about six months after treatment, you should be tested again six months after you stop taking aminoglycoside antibiotics.

The risk of hearing loss varies by the exact aminoglycoside antibiotic used. For example, amikacin is more ototoxic than gentamicin, but gentamicin is somewhat more likely to cause dizziness or balance problems. Erythromycin, very rarely impairs hearing. However, when it does, it's generally temporary. The physician participating in treatment must monitor hearing very carefully so permanent hearing loss in the frequency range needed to understand speech can be prevented.

As with chemotherapy patients, noise exposure during, and six months after, treatment is not recommended. If you develop any signs of hearing loss, dizziness, or tinnitus, your physician should be contacted. With aminoglycosides, the chance of a hearing loss is less than with cisplatin, and the chances are greater that you can be switched to another antibiotic if need be. Sometimes you'll be switched to another aminoglycoside antibiotic which is less ototoxic.

Keep in mind that if you take aminoglycoside antibiotics, keep a record of it because you'll be more vulnerable to hearing loss if you take them again in the future. Your physician will want to know which drug and how much of it you had in the previous treatment.

Antibiotic Eardrops and Ear Infections

Eardrops are generally quite safe. If you're prone to "swimmer's ear," or get other infections in your ear canals, your physician may prescribe antibiotic eardrops. But before prescribing, your physician should look in your ear to make sure that you don't have a hole in the eardrum. Many antibiotic eardrops contain an aminoglycoside antibiotic called neomycin which is very safe in the ear canal and on the eardrum. However, if you have a hole in your eardrum, particularly a large one, as can occur in a severe ear infection when the eardrum ruptures, the eardrops could go past the eardrum into the middle ear. In this case, the neomycin could make contact with the round window of the inner ear and cause hearing loss. While this is uncommon, it's important to have medical consultation if you get an ear infection rather than simply using the eardrops you used last time, or borrowing someone else's. Different ear infections need to be treated in different ways. Using the wrong type could make matters worse.

Over-the-Counter Drugs

Most of us will never experience any hearing problem from taking over-the-counter drugs. Most of the problems begin when patients start taking more than the recommended dose. "More is better" frequently does not apply to medications. When patients come to see me for hearing loss and/or tinnitus, one of my first questions is which drugs they are taking, particularly over-the-counter ones which may not be listed in their medical history. I'm often surprised at the number of people who assume that over-the-counter drugs have no side effects.

Loop Diuretics

Loop diuretics are used for congestive heart failure and other conditions to clear fluid. In adults, they sometimes temporarily impair hearing; there's some evidence that they can cause permanent hearing loss in newborns. We need additional research in order to draw more definitive conclusions. The main problem occurs if loop diuretics are given at the same time as an aminoglycoside antibiotic or cisplatin. This drug combination can cause severe and permanent hearing loss. Pharmacists and physicians are well aware of these interactions and conscientiously avoid them. The point is to be sure that your physician and pharmacist are always aware of *all* the drugs you're taking, even if it doesn't seem to be important to you at the time.

Hearing Loss Induced by Environmental Toxins

Sometimes we forget that our general health is related to the water we drink, and the air we breathe, but this is true for many aspects of our health including hearing loss. The people at greatest risk are those in jobs that expose them to chemicals on a daily basis. For these workers, it may be wise to get an annual hearing test. Industries naturally want to protect their workers, but standards for protecting hearing in these workers are not always well defined. For those of you looking for more information, Rybak (1992) offers a thorough scientific review in this area.

Trichloroethylene has been shown to cause hearing and balance problems which may be an early indication of toxicity in workers exposed to this chemical. Triethylchlorine is frequently used in grease removers, dry cleaning agents, spot removers, rug cleaners, and in making paints, waxes, pesticides, adhesives, and lubricants. For most of us who don't work with these chemicals on a daily basis, the risk of hearing or balance problems from them is quite low. However, always read labels carefully and if it states to use the agent in a well-ventilated area, take it seriously.

Xylene is found in many paints, varnishes, thinners, and is used in some laboratories; and **Styrene** is used in the production of plastics, synthetic rubbers, resins, and various insulating materials. These agents may cause actual hearing loss or can possibly make you less capable of understanding in difficult listening situations.

Hexane, a solvent used in many industries including shoe factories, doesn't necessarily impair hearing in the way we usually think of it; that is, an inability to hear soft sounds. Instead, hexane is neurotoxic—it can poison the nervous system including that part of the nervous system responsible for hearing, but the symptoms may be subtle and are not yet clearly defined. One symptom may be a decreased ability to perceive continuous tones (Bachmann et al. 1993) but more research needs to be done in this area.

Carbon disulfide is used in the viscose rayon process and as a solvent or insecticide. Like hexane, it's neurotoxic. However, carbon disulfide also appears to cause hearing loss and balance disorders.

Toluene is in the air we breathe because it's contained in motor vehicle and some industrial emissions. In industry, toluene is used in manufacturing chemicals, paints, lacquers, adhesives, rubber, some printing, and leather tanning. Toluene alone can occasionally damage hearing, but more commonly it seems to increase the amount of hearing loss caused by noise exposure, so hearing protection around noise is even more important for these workers. Toluene also seems to affect the portion of the brain responsible for processing and understanding sound. It's also found in some home products. So again, always follow label instructions and use in a well-ventilated area whenever indicated.

Incidentally, the combination of some of these chemicals with noise exposure greatly increases the odds of hearing loss. Therefore, if the risk of noise-induced hearing loss in industries using these chemicals is higher than in other industries, and if you use these chemicals at home while using power tools, be extra careful about wearing hearing protection.

Carbon Monoxide Poisoning, either deliberate as in suicide attempts or accidental as in industrial or home accidents, can cause hearing loss. Sometimes, but not always, the hearing partially or completely recovers. Carbon monoxide can not only affect the hearing itself but the brain pathways that conduct and process the auditory signals. Hopefully, you already have a carbon monoxide detector in your home. They are very inexpensive and available at most hardware stores. However, if you or someone you know is poisoned by carbon monoxide, be sure and get a hearing test too.

Heavy Metals including arsenic, mercury, tin, manganese, and lead can all affect the auditory system. Certainly no one would deliberately expose themselves to these metals, but nonetheless, unintentional exposure can occur in a number of ways. For example, arsenic occurs in soils and ores. In one case in the 1970s, a coal-burning plant used coal containing arsenic and thus released air borne arsenic which caused hearing loss in people living near the plant (Bencko & Symon 1977). In the 1950s, Japan reported an outbreak of a new disease called "Minamata Disease" (it occurred around Minamata, Japan). Eighty percent of these people developed hearing loss and other problems including numbness in their limbs, visual impairments, a drunken walk, and a host of other conditions. Most of them either died or were left with severe permanent disability (Kurland et al., 1960). As discussed by Rybak (1992), similar problems were found in patients in the mid 1960s in Japan and in the 1970s in Iraq. The underlying culprit was found to be industrial mercury contaminating the food supply either through fish, shellfish, or grain.

Lead seems to be everywhere in the environment. Leaded gasoline has accounted for most of the lead in air pollution. Unfortunately, by the time we switched to "unleaded," the lead had already been absorbed by the water, soil, and plants in our environment.

Substance Abuse and Hearing Loss

Unfortunately, some of the previously listed industrial chemicals can be used to get "high." Xylene, toluene, hexane, various organic solvents, and butyl nitrite (used in some air fresheners) are sometimes "sniffed." However, as just described, the substance abuser may also receive permanent hearing loss and in some cases the auditory nerves, brain stem, and brain are affected which gives you an idea of the general damage that can occur.

Many times we don't know as much as we'd like about the consequences of substance abuse because the abusers are such a difficult group to study. It's very difficult to document how much of the chemical the person received, how long they've been using it, what other substances they also use. Because these activities are illegal, they're usually hidden. Also, street drugs are often "cut" with other substances, so the exact content is usually unknown. Marijuana and caffeine have been implicated as possibly causing tinnitus or making it worse if you do have it (Schulman 1991). But then nicotine (Meyerhoff & Mickey 1988), and alcohol consumption (Quaranta et al., 1996), have also been implicated.

Preventing Ear Infections

Ear infections are very common in children but adults get them too. There are some things we can do to reduce their likelihood. Reducing or eliminating smoking can decrease the chances of upper respiratory infections including ear infections. Remaining free of other irritants, like constant wood smoke exposure, can also decrease the risk of ear infections.

Part II: Preventing Noise-and Music-Induced Hearing Loss

The amount of hearing loss one might receive from noise depends on its intensity, the amount of time you're exposed to it, and to a lesser extent it's frequency. All of these things are difficult to measure and document for recreational noise. Noise-induced hearing loss usually affects high frequencies. Also, individual susceptibility varies so greatly. The same noise which doesn't damage hearing in one person, may cause substantial hearing loss in someone standing next to him and we don't completely understand this. Certainly some differences may be attributable to the angle of the noise, the reverberation in a particular location, the person's body position, and so forth, but we're only beginning to understand the influence of genetic predisposition, diet, general health, smoking, and a number of other factors.

While we expect very loud noise to cause pain, levels well below this can result in permanent hearing loss, devoid of pain, particularly over a period of time. If all noise that could damage your hearing caused pain, perhaps we'd know to avoid it. But since it doesn't hurt and sometimes we even welcome it, as in loud music at concerts, it's deceptively dangerous. Overall, if it's so loud that you have to raise your voice to easily carry on a conversation, consider yourself at risk.

Noise as a Stressor

High noise levels not only cause hearing loss, but they can evoke a stress response in the body. Some people like this stress response. For example, in aerobics classes, the music level is deliberately kept high to give participants "more energy." In concerts, the stress response causes a feeling of excitement and jubilation.

Studies of populations that are not exposed to noise, (like remote tribes in the Sudan and Easter Island), don't experience hearing loss with aging. While these remote populations also have other differences including a high-fiber low-fat diet, virtually no obesity, no industrial pollutants, lots of exercise, and genetic differences, there's good reason to suspect that some of the hearing loss that we've associated with aging may actually be at least partially a result of accumulated noise exposure over years.

Implications of Noise

Typically, the onset of noise-induced hearing loss is very slow and subtle, although a loud blast injury may cause a sudden drop in hearing. You may notice a bit more difficulty in understanding speech in noisy listening environments or have more trouble with children and women's voices than with men's voices. In this very early stage, the hearing health care provider may tell you that there's a "noise notch" in your audiogram which is an *early warning sign*. What this means is that hearing at one or two of the high frequencies (usually around 4000 to 6000 Hz) has diminished, while hearing at other frequencies may still be very good. In fact, hearing at 4000 Hz may still technically be within the "normal" range but the fact that it is slightly worse at just one or two high frequencies reveals that unless you protect yourself, it will probably get worse.

The incidence of "noise notches" in professional musicians has been found to range as high as 90 percent. Also, while the noise levels and hearing protection programs in industry are carefully regulated and monitored, noise exposure of many professional musicians frequently exceeds that of industrial workers. However, many musicians, who depend on their hearing for their livelihood, do not routinely obtain hearing tests or use hearing protection. A little self-education might pay off.*

Like hunters, many times musicians will have hearing loss worse

*See Reference listing for Chasin, a useful resource on noise education and hearing protection if you're a musician.

in one ear because the intensity of the sound is greater on one side. For example, right-handed violinists may have poorer hearing on the left side because the sound is generated closest to that side. Conversely, right-handed flute players may have poorer hearing on the right side for the same reason. Most types of noise exposure cause peak loss of hearing around 4000 Hz. However, in musicians, especially those who play only one type of instrument, the frequency of loss is often related to the type of instrument they play. For example, a piccolo player may have damaged hearing in a higher frequency range than a drummer. Unfortunately, this means that the loss will generally be worse in the frequency range that the musician needs most! However, this does not mean that the cello player will have a low frequency hearing loss and the piccolo player will have a high frequency hearing loss. For several reasons, the high frequency portion of the ear is more vulnerable to any type of noise exposure. Therefore, regardless of the type of noise, hearing loss is generally worse at high frequencies. Tinnitus can often accompany any type of high frequency hearing loss, particularly when noise-induced.

Interestingly, there's research which suggests that if you dislike the music, your risk for damaged hearing increases (and regrettably, liking the music will not protect your hearing). As reviewed by Chasin (1996), several different studies have shown this in different ways. Technicians who dislike the music they're working around tend to receive greater hearing loss than musicians who enjoy it. This difference may be due to the effects of stress which change hormonal levels in the people who really dislike the music. A positive way of looking at this is to feel reassured about walking out on a concert you don't like!

Another problem which can develop, especially to professional musicians, is called *diplacusis*. When this occurs, the musician may no longer perceive pitch correctly. In fact, when a musical note gets higher in frequency, the musician may think that the pitch is the same but the loudness has changed. Obviously, this can be a major problem for musicians. Once this happens, the damage cannot be corrected, although proper hearing protection can ward off further insult.

In the meantime, we have to put more effort into preventing noise- and music-induced hearing loss because once it occurs, it's generally permanent. Sometimes, people are misled because they'll notice decreased hearing or experience tinnitus after noise or music exposure which is often followed by some improvement over the next day or two. Unfortunately, what usually happens is that the hearing never returns to the original level. The very delicate hair cell structures inside the inner ear become weakened and die off. And you become much more vulnerable to future damage from noise, drugs, or fevers.

Who's at Risk?

One of the most frustrating things for hearing health care providers is that we see so much noise- and music- induced hearing loss which could be prevented. Unfortunately, we don't usually see people until after their hearing is impaired, and by then, it's too late. Some people, particularly musicians and music fans, resent calling hearing loss caused by loud music "noise-induced." But for the purposes of this chapter the term "noise" will be used to refer to any loud sound including music.

Musicians and Concert-Goers

Music-induced hearing loss is more commonly observed in professional musicians than in concert-goers because musicians are exposed to noise for longer periods of time. Most research regarding hearing loss and professional musicians has been carried out on them in symphonies and concert bands. They're easier to study because they more commonly perform in the same or similar environment each time, and data collection is easier on a large group of people with similar noise exposure. Rock musicians have been less well-studied because they tend to perform in small groups, in varying environments, and tend to be an independent breed who are not always concerned about their hearing. However, there's good reason to believe that rock musicians may be at even greater risk of hearing loss than symphony musicians because the music and audience tend to be louder and the noise level tends to remain at a high level throughout the concert.

If noise-induced damage is so common in professional musicians, it may be questioned, why they don't notice it early-on? One reason is that this type of hearing loss usually happens very slowly. Because musicians don't notice a sudden change, they gradually adapt to the way things sound without even noticing any compensating mechanism. Another reason is that in the early stages at high intensity levels, music will often sound the same as before. It's only at soft levels that the difference will first become noticeable. By the time a musician notices problems, the condition may be somewhat advanced. For this reason, professional musicians should have annual hearing tests and use carefully selected hearing protectors.

Firearm Users

Hunters and other firearm users frequently suffer permanent hearing loss, often accompanied by tinnitus. In fact, it's been estimated that over 50 percent of shooters and hunters are hearing impaired as a result of firearm noise levels. Usually, the hearing loss is worse at high frequencies, and is worse on the ear opposite the side on which you hold the gun. The major impact of the gun's blast is greatest on the opposite side because the output of the barrel is closest to that side. So don't be surprised if you tell your hearing health care provider that you're a hunter, you're asked whether you're right- or left-handed!

There are several types of hearing protectors available for use with firearms (See Figure 12-1). The military and other work environments that require firearm use like the Federal Bureau of Investigation, the police, the Drug Enforcement Agency, and so forth, all have to follow strict guidelines for hearing protection and noise control. Sometimes, I have patients from the military who tell me they remove one earplug whenever they're listening for firing commands. For these individuals, I recommend the hunters earplugs as described later.

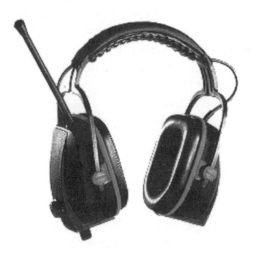

[Photo Courtesy of Dalloz Safety]

Figure 12-1: Earmuff Protector (with wireless listening capability, such as a radio or telecommunication). You need to know what your sound exposure levels are in order to know which earmuff would be best for your needs. Most of these earmuffs cover a range of protection between 125 Hz and 8,000 Hz. Their peak attenuation can reach as high as 29 dB, but can exceed this if you wear protective earplugs in conjunction with the earmuff.

226

The popularity of target practice ranges, trap shoots, and self-protection firearms programs has increased. The output of a firearm is so intense that some people get permanent hearing loss from only one or two exposures. Be sure to obtain high quality, high attenuation (dampening) hearing protectors for these environments. If you get earmuffs, which are frequently recommended for high attenuation protection, be sure that they fit you perfectly and that they do not have even a pinhole leak or gap around your face or glasses. Nowadays, earmuff protectors even come with a variety of built-in options, such as wireless communication devices or piped-in music.

Industrial Workers

OSHA regulations specify allowable noise levels and length of noise exposure in industrial environments. They also dictate how often workers should have hearing tests and the type of hearing protection used. If you work in one of these environments, naturally you need to follow all of these guidelines to protect your hearing. If you loosen your hearing protectors because they're uncomfortable or remove them because you feel you don't hear well enough with them, your risk goes up.

Recreational Participants

With respect to the hazards of recreational noise, little research has been conducted. Noise control and protection standards for industry are somewhat difficult to apply to other situations because such standards are for an eight-hour exposure five days per week. How does this compare to the person with little noise exposure at work but who then rides a motorcycle home and goes to rock concerts twice a month? Or what about the office worker whose hobby is woodworking? Unlike the industrial environment, it's very difficult to study the effects of this type of noise exposure because it's so variable.

There are so many recreational noise sources that it's not practical to list them here. I use the term "recreational" loosely. I realize that not everyone considers mowing the lawn or remodeling the bathroom to be recreational activity. Some retirees have more noise exposure from their retirement activities than they did on their job. How great is your risk from developing hearing loss because of your non-work exposure? It actually depends on a number of factors including how often you're exposed to the noise, the intensity of the noise, and whether the noise is steady or intermittent. However, even if we consider all these factors, we still could not exactly predict how much hearing loss you may receive. It may depend on your genetics and whether people in your family are prone to hearing loss; whether you have blue or brown eyes (some people think that blue-eyed people are at greater risk although anyone can get noise-induced hearing loss); which types of medications you're taking or have taken in the past; and possibly if you have had your auditory system weakened by previous exposure to certain environmental toxins, viruses, diseases, or fevers.

Other Professionals

Some work environments are not routinely monitored by OSHA but nonetheless can expose workers to undesirable noise levels. Dentists, dental assistants, gardeners, mechanics, race car drivers and their pit crews, construction workers, metal workers, farmers, wood workers, aerobic instructors, emergency vehicle drivers, carpet cleaners and so forth, may be exposed to noise, and yet may not be informed about the need for hearing protection, particularly if they have their own business or work for a small company. Sometimes, the actual risk of hearing loss is difficult to document because the noise is intermittent and varies so much from one work environment to the next. Fortunately, many industrial plants have charts listing the best type of hearing protection for each of these professions. Your hearing care provider can work with them in selecting the best hearing protection for you.

Smoking, Diet and Fitness

We hear so much about the importance of getting more exercise, reducing fat in our diet, quitting smoking and so forth (Campbell et al., 1996). There seems to be a correlation between a high-fat diet and cardiovascular problems as we have all read about. Not surprisingly, there also seems to be a correlation between good health habits and preservation of hearing, although we have a great deal to learn about it. It's difficult to study patients over a number of years to determine which ones develop hearing loss. Several studies have also shown a correlation between a high-fat diet and hearing loss, and between cardiovascular problems and hearing loss, and between "lipid disorders" (loosely termed "cholesterol problems"), and hearing loss, although they may be all getting at the same issue. Not only can all of these problems cause or increase the likelihood of damaging hearing, but they seem to really increase the likelihood and amount of hearing loss in the presence of noise.

A high-fat diet and poor cardiovascular fitness appear to increase your risk of hearing loss. Conversely, physically fit people tend to be more resistant to noise-induced hearing loss. Furthermore, as indicated earlier, there's some evidence that exercising in the presence of noise may even increase the probability of incurring hearing loss (Vittitow et al., 1994). So, you might want to wear earplugs or ask your aerobics instructor to turn down the music.

Also as mentioned earlier, keep in mind that smoking has some harmful effects on hearing. It decreases the oxygen and blood supply to the inner ear. It also increases the level of carbon monoxide. These factors not only can impair hearing, but smokers are more prone to noise-induced hearing loss.

Prevention and Protection

Contrary to popular belief, cotton balls are not an effective form of hearing protection. In fact, cotton is not a good idea because it can leave debris in the ear canal, attracting dirt and possibly infection. Effective hearing protection is available in the form of plugs or earmuffs. For some very noisy environments, earmuffs and earplugs can be jointly worn. The benefit of earmuffs is that in addition to protection from sound traveling through the ear canal, a portion of the side of the head where the high frequency area of the cochlear is most exposed and vulnerable, there is added protection.

A Word of Caution

Earmuffs and earplugs have ratings on the package so you can compare them. Frequently, the protection provided by each hearing protector is listed as the "attenuation." In general, the greater the attenuation, the more effective the hearing protection. Sometimes, the amount of attenuation is listed according to a variety of rating schemes which categorize each protector into a single classification. These categorizations can get very complicated and can vary from country to country, so you might want to have your hearing health care provider help you. When you shop for earplugs, be sure they're designed for *hearing protection*. Sometimes people buy earplugs designed to keep water out of the ears or to protect the ear against pressure changes rather than for noise exposure. Some patients assume that if they turn off their hearing aids, they can double as hearing protectors, but hearing aids are not designed to reduce noise. If your hearing aid is vented, it will not adequately protect your hearing from noise even when it's turned off.

Many earplugs are specially designed for different types of listening needs. Musicians can order special plugs which reduce the overall level of sound but without distorting it (See Chapter 13). In fact, there are different plugs recommended for musicians who play different types of musical instruments. Concert-goers often can enjoy musician's plugs as well.

References

Bachmann, M.O., DeBeer, S. and Myers, J.E. N-hexane neurotoxicity in metal can manufacturing workers. Occupational Medicine, Vol. 43 (3), 149-154, 1993.

Bencko, V. and Symon, K. Test of environmental exposure to arsenic and hearing changes in exposed children. Environmental Health Perspectives, Vol. 13, 386-395, 1977.

Campbell, K. Ototoxicity: current issues. American Journal of Audiology, Vol.2 (1), 15-16, 1993.

Campbell, K. and Durrant, J. Audiologic monitoring for ototoxicity. The Otolaryngologic Clinics of North America, Vol. 26, 903-914, 1993.

Campbell, K., Rybak, L. and Khadori, R. Sensorineural hearing loss and dyslipidemia. American Journal of Audiology, Vol. 5 (3), 11-14, 1996.

Chasin, M. Musicians and the Prevention of Hearing Loss. San Diego:Singular Publishing, 1996.

Dobie, R.A. Noise-induced hearing loss and acoustic trauma. Medical-Legal Evaluation of Hearing Loss. New York: Van Nostand Reinhold, 1993.

Jung, T., Rhee, C., Lee, C., Park, Y. and Choi, D. Ototoxicity of salicylate, nonsteroidal anti-inflammatory drugs and quinine. In The Otolaryngologic Clinics of North America, L. P. Rybak, (Ed.), Vol. 26 (5), 791-810, 1993.

Kurland, L. T., Faro, S. N. and Siedler, H. Minamata disease: the outbreak of a neurologic disorder in Minamata, Japan, and its relationship to the ingestion of seafood contaminated by mercuric compounds. World Neurology Vol. 1, 370-395, 1960.

Meyerhoff, W. L. and Mickey, B. E. Vascular decompression of the cochlear nerve in tinnitus sufferers. Laryngoscope, Vol. 98 (5 pt. 1), 602-604, 1988.

Quaranta, A., Assennato, G. and Sallustio, V. Epidemiology of hearing problems among adults in Italy. Scandinavian Audiology, (supplementum), Vol. 42, 9-13, 1996.

Rybak, L. P. Hearing: the effects of chemicals. Otolaryngology- Head and Neck Surgery, Vol. 106 (6), 677-686, 1992.

Schulman, A. Medical methods, drug therapy, and tinnitus control strategies. Tinnitus, pp. 453-489, Philadelphia: Lea & Febiger, 1991.

Vittitow M., Windmill I. M., Yates J. W. and Cunningham, D.R. Effect of simultaneous exercise and noise exposure (music) on hearing. Journal of the American Academy of Audiology, Vol. 5 (5), 343-348, 1994.

Introduction

Section IV: Products and Resources

Paula Bonillas
Editor, *Hearing Health*
Ingleside, Texas

I vividly remember my search years ago for something more than hearing aids that might help me as I struggled with my declining hearing. Already wearing the strongest behind-the-ear hearing aids on the market, I knew I needed more. But what?

The answer came over time—assistive listening devices (ALDs) and contact with others like myself. My quest began 15 years ago when I literally stumbled across a small, portable telephone amplifier that changed my life. For the first time in many years, I could use the telephone while away from my home. If I was running late for an appointment, my portable amplifier enabled me to use a pay phone. No longer forced to be telephone-dependent, I was spurred to continue searching for more products. It was the discovery of ALDs that motivated me to change careers in mid-stream and launch *Hearing Health* magazine.

The lack of available information about assistive devices surprised me, especially given the tremendous boost they provided, not only to communication but to my morale as well. It became my mission in life to share the information I found. So, naturally, I was delighted when I was invited to write an Introduction to this section.

The field of assistive listening devices has literally exploded in the past 15 years. Every week, I receive releases about new products that are coming onto the market. In this technological age, it's a very difficult to keep abreast of the latest products, to list everything available today would take an entire book.

Knowing what would work best for you may be confusing at first. Ask your hearing health care professional to advise you, especially with the enhanced listening devices. Some of these products work better with certain types of hearing aids, and are better suited for particular types of hearing loss. Simply having a telecoil in your hearing aid can often make a tremendous difference when selecting listening devices. If your hearing aids don't have a telecoil, ask your provider about adding this option. Many people can benefit from them, and installing one is relatively inexpensive. A number of ALDs are much easier to use and are ultimately less expensive when a telecoil is already included in the hearing aid.

Naturally, some manufacturers and distributors are more than happy to guide you, but many are not accessible by the public. Nevertheless, if you're so inclined to explore these products, before long you'll have a communication-equipped house, car, boat, church, workplace—life! If you're like me, you may have a tendency to go overboard at first. In the beginning, I had all the bells and whistles. Flashing lights and loud bells throughout the house alerted me that the telephone or doorbell was ringing—still a rather shocking experience for unaware guests when the phone rings! I was "wired" with induction loops for communication in every room. Infrared was installed for my television set, along with a captioning decoder. And for away-from-home insurance, I carried a portable FM system.

In addition to ALDs, it was contact with organizations and people who understood and accepted my communication woes that kept my boat afloat. The organizations and resources listed in this section are invaluable. Answers to questions about everything from how to get captions on your television to what can be done about tinnitus can be obtained through these contacts. But most importantly, you'll realize that you're not alone. Indeed, in the U.S., some 28 million others are struggling in varying degrees with the same problems you are. Many of those, but not nearly enough, have joined self-help groups to share insights, difficulties and coping strategies with each another.

Ironically, the problems that beset people with hearing impairment are the ones that keep them from joining groups like Self Help for Hard of Hearing People (SHHH). The tendency to remain in self-imposed isolation may be almost overwhelming, but that's obviously not a healthy choice. Making that first contact is a critical first step. If there are no groups in your area—start one. Undoubtedly, others will benefit. The organizations will guide you in every way the can.

It's amazing to watch people who come to these meetings for the first time. A metamorphosis takes place because self-help groups are "safe." People who might otherwise sit silently in fear that they might say something that has absolutely nothing to do with the topic begin to share their problems and ask openly for assistance. Every person's unique communication needs are taken into account. I've seen less technologically advanced groups use an overhead projector with a note-taker writing during the entire meeting to ensure that everyone is understanding. Most groups, however, are more apt to offer hands-on opportunities to try various types of assistive equipment and will offer listening devices you can use to boost your hearing aids during the meetings. Some more advanced groups even have real-time captioning during their meetings.

The saddest thing a hard of hearing or late-deafened person can do is nothing. If hearing aids are not enough, then your life suffers. Certainly, no mechanical devices are a panacea for the hearing we once had, or the hearing we might hope to have, but ALDs are indispensable. They keep us "connected" with others. Review the following pages carefully. It can be a new way of thinking about communication. When you take this first crucial step, whether it's asking your hearing health care professional about assistive devices, or contacting an organization for membership, you'll find yourself, once again, in control of your life.

CHAPTER THIRTEEN

From Hearing Aids to Assistive Listening Devices [ALDs]

Richard Carmen, Au.D.

Fewer than 20 years ago, for consumers with impaired hearing, there were very limited choices of alternative amplification devices other than hearing aids. In the 1970s, most telephone amplification equipment was issued at no charge to accounts under American Telephone and Telegraph companies. However, since "Ma Bell's" break-up, a tremendous flood of market possibilities has opened up for new companies and products. This is a great boon to all who have hearing loss, as the rather fierce competition for this narrow market keeps the prices of these products affordable.

Something which has probably not yet occurred, although the trend is moving in this direction, is the general acceptance among audiologists and hearing instrument specialists that there is tremendous value in other devices besides hearing aids. This doesn't mean instead of hearing aids, but whatever equipment can augment, enhance, or for the duration of the experience, improve listening and hearing. For some, this will mean a television headset for amplification fulfillment without the momentary need of wearing hearing aids. For others, it may mean a telephone amplifier with or without a hearing aid. And still others may benefit from a special telephone designed for use with the optional "T" coil in a hearing aid. Many of these devices can take the edge off hearing difficulties, and in some cases, even fully solve the problem. Something as simple as not blasting the television (by having your own remote amplifier) has solved many an argument and household disruption. Whatever your specific requirements, the purpose of this chapter is to bring your attention to the great variety of augmentative amplifying choices you have. These products should give you a good overview, and you should understand that there are many variations on the same theme, one of which may nicely fit your personal needs. Perhaps by seeing some of these, you'll be inspired to take advantage of them, or further explore such possibilities.

In the event that your provider does not handle ALDs, you may request that he or she become familiar with these products and companies and consider carrying them, or at least have them available to order. On the other hand, I must caution you that many hearing health care professionals are simply too busy to handle adding ALDs to their practice. In this case, you could at least request some names of companies that might deal directly with consumers.

There are a number of companies that manufacture or distribute very similar devices, particularly in the area of alarm clocks, television amplifying equipment, and telephone ringer-amplified and receiver-amplified products. For example, for standard telephone receiver handsets, several items are available to clip over the earpiece of the receiver to allow you significant audio boost on incoming calls. Such "portability" allows you to carry this in your pocket wherever you go and use it on any telephone when you travel. Others are built into the receiver handset and are sold as a single unit which replaces your current receiver. And still others are manufactured by connection to your telephone line and provide amplification this way. Naturally, there are a variety of prices, depending on which product you select from a particular company.

Every primary U.S. manufacturer* and distributor* was contacted and invited to participate in this chapter. They were asked to provide a photograph and description of one product they carry or manufacture. It's not important for you to differentiate between who manufactures and who is strictly a distributor. In fact, some manufacturers also do their own distribution (as well as carrying other companies' products). The names of the companies cited as having provided a photo courtesy of their organization was done to allow hearing health care professionals who might not be familiar with these devices and companies, to have an opportunity to contact them and establish an in-house corner of their office to display some of them. They'll need to know that most distributors carry a variety of the products listed here.

*Based on listings which appeared in the Worldwide Registry published by The Hearing Review, Vol. 4., No.5, May, 1997.

Listing manufacturers and distributors for your convenience and familiarity in this chapter in no way should be construed as an endorsement of any company or device by the publisher, the editor or any contributing authors of this book. Any purchase of these devices is a responsibility between you and the company from which you make the purchase. Also, it's important for you to bear in mind that these products were not rated in any way. That is, it cannot be assumed that a particular product listed here is any better or worse than a comparable item not listed here.

Finally, something of importance you should know is what warranty coverage you have on particular products. For example, some items carry only a 90-day warranty while others, a variation on the same theme, can have one year. Some products have as much as a five-year warranty. Some companies have specific requirements for returns, and may charge you a "restocking fee." Make these inquiries *before you make the purchase*. Prices have been purposely excluded because they can so easily change. However, you should know that most of these devices are reasonably under $100, and the few that aren't are essentially under $300 each, as of this printing.

Products are listed alphabetically within each category by the company who provided the photo.

Alerting Devices

Wireless Personal Pager
is a vibrating sensor that alerts you up to 100 feet away that someone wants your attention. This battery operated device can be used in the office, around the house, or outdoors. It can also be utilized if bedridden. Activation occurs through the push of a button.

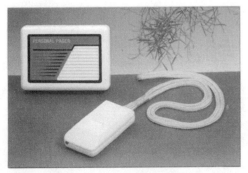

[Photo Courtesy of Hear More, Inc.]

Vibrating Wristwatch
is a multi-purpose watch that can be preset to a specific time to vibrate and remind you to take your medication, attend a meeting, make a phone call, and so forth. It comes with an audio alarm setting as well. Additional features include stop watch function, four countdown timer functions with an LCD indicator, worldwide time in 24 cities, a three second auto-off backlight, and includes long life lithium batteries.

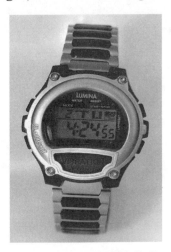

[Photo Courtesy of LS&S Group]

Watchman Signaling System

is an alerting system which consists of various options you can add to fit your personal needs. For example, the Phone Master directly connects to your phone line to flash a lamp for incoming calls; the Doorbell Master will alert you to someone at the door; the Sound Master can alert you to a baby crying, or other important sounds.

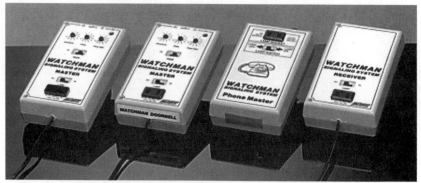

[Photo Courtesy of Potomac Technologies, Inc.]

Shake-Up Smoke Detector Kit

has a loud 85 dB horn (at 10 feet), with a radius up to a 125 feet. The system is battery powered, and 3" by 5." Options include a strobe light, or vibrating alert by means of an internal thermal switch.

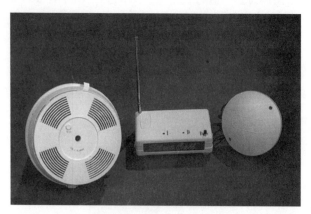

[Photo Courtesy of Silent Call Corporation]

Automotive Devices

Siren Alert

is an emergency vehicle detection system that allows drivers of any vehicle to know that a fire truck, police car, ambulance or other emergency vehicle is approaching (even when out of sight). It is portable, sits on the dashboard, and should be hard-wired to the ignition switch. The company states that the V.A. will make full reimbursement to all veterans who have established service connection for hearing loss. It is effective up to 500 feet away from the signaling source. Cigarette lighter power source. NOTE: This system will not detect emergency vehicle *air horns,* and on occasion, will false-detect.

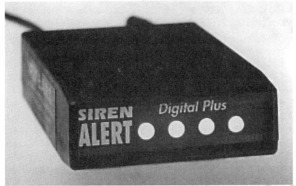

[Photo Courtesy of EARS Systems, Inc.]

Blinker Buddy: Electronic Turn Signal Reminder

alerts you to the turn signal being on by flashing a light and sounding an alert. The longer the turn signal remains on, the louder the volume. The volume resets when the brake is pressed. The hard-wired installation may require a mechanic.

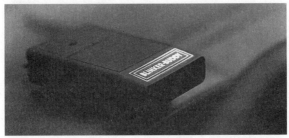

[Photo Courtesy of HARC Mercantile Ltd.]

Enhanced Listening Devices

Sound Wizard

is a personal communication device with a directional microphone that allows you to hear better in the presence of background noises such as in restaurants, meetings, and so forth.

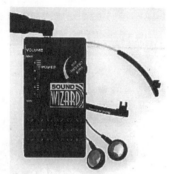

[Photo Courtesy of Hitec Group International, Inc.]

Listening Glass II

is a portable high fidelity stereo sound amplifier usable in particularly noisy environments. It comes with rechargeable batteries capable of full charge overnight.

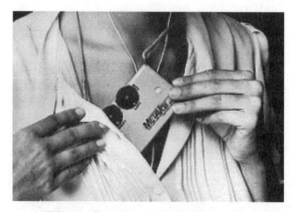

[Photo Courtesy of Metavox, Inc.]

ProPhonic IV Professional Earphone Monitor (for musicians)
is a professional earphone that houses modular drivers in precision custom earmolds. It functions as both a hearing protection device as well as a live monitor that permits high frequency extension. It allows a performer to hear the full dynamic range of music without feedback or exposure to ear-shattering sound levels. Cords and transducers (extras of which are not included) are easily replaceable.

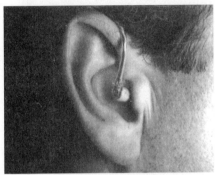

[Photo Courtesy of Sensaphonics, Inc.]

Pocketalker Pro
is a battery operated portable amplifier designed to improve your ability to communicate in difficult listening situations, such as noisy environments (achieved by the microphone being placed next to the person speaking). The unit has a sensitive directional microphone with an extension cord for television listening, and the amplifier is compact with a volume control. It comes with a belt clip and a carrying case. Also, you have an option of an earpiece, earphone or headphone. The unit may also be used with your hearing aid, or in conjunction with the telephone (requires additional telephone adapter).

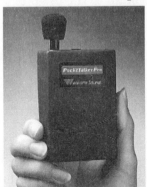

[Photo Courtesy of Williams
Sound Corporation]

241

Telephone Devices

Ameriphone Super Phone Ringer

is one of the loudest ringers (up to 95 dB) for people who have difficulty hearing their telephone ring, especially from a distance. It plugs into a modular jack, has adjustable tone and volume control, and can be desk- or wall-mounted.

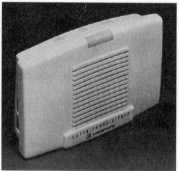

[Photo Courtesy of Adco
Hearing Products, Inc.]

Tel-Ease Telephone

comes in variable tone ringers depending on your hearing loss, for ease in hearing the telephone ring. The three ranges are 550 Hz, 1250 Hz, or 2,000 Hz. The volume is adjustable up to 95 dBA. It is hearing aid compatible, has 10-number memory, and automatic redial. It has two special features: a Back-Talk is a voice synthesized dialing aid that actually repeats audibly the number that has been dialed (to protect against dialing the wrong number), and a Data Jack feature allows an additional device to hook up to the telephone line, such as a computer.

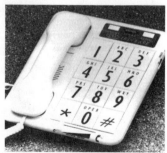

[Photo Courtesy of Communication
Products and Equipment Company]

AT&T Answering Machine Model 1721M

allows you to hear and understand your messages more clearly by listening with headphones, a neckloop, silhouette, direct audio input, or even a cochlear implant adapter cord. It has all the primary features of an answering machine including LED display of number of calls, two-way call recording, call screening and remote access.

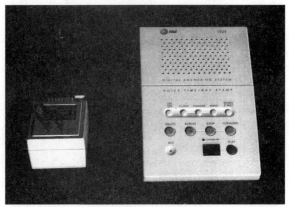

[Photo Courtesy of General Technologies]

Portable Telephone Amplifier

merely straps over the earpiece of any telephone handset receiver and allows you adjustment of the volume of incoming voices. Operates on batteries and is hearing aid compatible. Usable on any telephone.

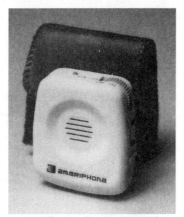

[Photo Courtesy of
Hal-Hen Company]

Walker Clarity Phone W-1000
has a slide bar that allows increased volume for high frequencies to improve the clarity of what you hear. The ringer bell has three different pitch options to accommodate various hearing losses. The receiver is hearing aid compatible. It also has a visual ring indicator.

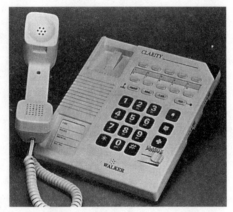

[Photo Courtesy of Harris
Communications, Inc.]

Uniphone 1140
is a combination TTY, telephone and amplified handset all in one. This unit increases volume up to 20 dB, includes 8k memory for conversation review and auto-answer, auto-answer messages, keyboard dial, 10-speed dial keys, and last number redial. A printer port is included to use with an external printer. Caller ID is a standard feature.

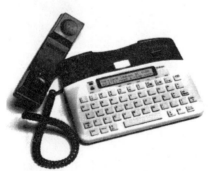

[Photo Courtesy of Ultratec Inc.]

Cordless Amplified Telephone

has the volume control built into the handset which can be programmed and preset up to a 14 dB increase. The 25 channel selection allows you the flexibility to move around your home or office and still be in touch. Features include a 20-number memory autodial, Caller ID, Call Waiting, and rechargeable batteries. For an additional cost, a printer cable is available for connection to an external printer.

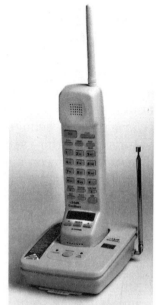

[Photo Courtesy of Weitbrecht Communications, Inc.]

Television

Closed Caption Decoder

allows viewers with hearing loss to view spoken dialogue as printed words on the television screen. Unlike subtitles, captions are specifically designed for deaf and hard of hearing viewers. Captions are capable of identifying speakers, on- and off-screen sound effects, music and laughter. Newer decoders now have an option which allows you to turn the captions on or off by the flick of a switch.

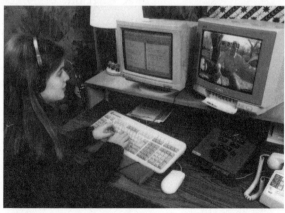

[Photo Courtesy of The Caption Center]

DirectEar Personal Listening System

is an infrared wireless system that provides the listener with complete, private and substantial audio amplification of the television, independent of the volume on the set itself. Therefore, it doesn't interfere with other people viewing or listening in the same room. It's also compatible with many infrared amplifying systems in movie theaters and other facilities. In fact, many

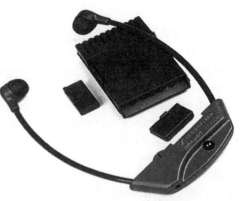

[Photo Courtesy of Sennheiser Electronic Corporation]

theaters will allow you to bring the headset with you. The system comes with one rechargeable battery. A second rechargeable battery is recommended so that you won't be inconvenienced from listening due to battery recharge time.

Wake-Up Devices

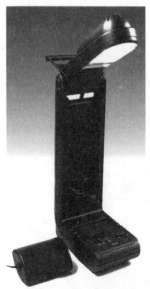

[Photo Courtesy of Global Assistive Devices, Inc.]

Access Alarm Clock

offers a variety of options and can minimize bedside clutter. It has the superior light of a halogen lamp, a clock with battery back-up, an LED display, and a snooze button. A telephone cord is supplied for hook-up to allow increased telephone ring intensity. The unit comes with an auxiliary jack for use with other company products.

Bed Vibrator

is recommended for heavy sleepers and designed for double, queen or king size beds. It allows a gentle but substantial vibration to be sent through the mattress to awaken the user.

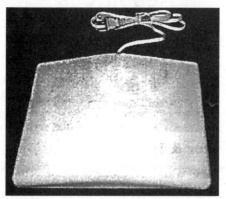

[Photo Courtesy of NFSS

Sonic Boom Alarm Clock

is designed to wake up very heavy sleepers. You can select any combination of modes to awaken to a loud pulsating audio alarm, flashing lights, or a shaking bed. The clock has large bright green numbers and a built-in receiver to pick up transmissions from other company products. An option at extra cost is a vibrator for the bed capable of producing pulsing or continuous patterns.

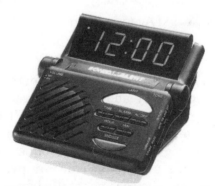

[Photo Courtesy of Sonic Alert]

CHAPTER FOURTEEN
Resources

There are many service organizations which offer information to consumers with impaired hearing. Some carry leaflets or brochures and others provide referral services. Some do not have any current consumer services but are cited here to allow you to write to them regarding questions you might have about a particular problem which you feel they might best address. Hopefully, this will give you the opportunity to expand your present search.

In the organizations' listings, besides telephone and address contacts, many have e-mail and website established. If you're on the Internet, you can access them directly. In the text that follows, background, company function, and their publications are included. If you're writing a request for information, I encourage you to enclose a self-addressed stamped business-size envelope large enough to accommodate your requested literature. If you're telephoning, especially on the toll free 800 numbers, please consider that many of these offices are in the east (E.S.T. zone), and some close by 4:00 p.m. Each call of course is a cost to them.

Academy of Dispensing Audiologists [ADA]
3008 Millwood Avenue, Columbia, SC 29205
Voice: (803) 252-5646 Fax: (803) 765-0860
E-mail:info@audiologist.org web:http://www.hear4U.com

Founded in 1977, the Academy supports the professional dispensing of hearing aids by audiologists in rehabilitative practice who have achieved a graduate degree in the field. They hold an annual meeting in the fall, and smaller regional meetings and seminars providing information regarding all aspects of hearing aid dispensing. *Feedback* is their quarterly magazine for professionals which addresses current issues. They are not staffed for consumer outreach.

Acoustic Neuroma Association [ANA]
P.O. Box 12402, Atlanta, GA 30355
Voice: (404) 237-8023 Fax: (404) 237-2704
E-mail:anausa@aol.com web:http://132.183.175.10/ana/m

The Acoustic Neuroma Association is a non-profit, patient-organized information and mutual-aid group, founded in 1981. They provide information and support to patients who have been diagnosed with or experienced an acoustic neuroma or other benign problems affecting the cranial nerves. They furnish information on patient rehabilitation to physicians and health care personnel, and promote and support research on acoustic neuroma and its effects. They educate the public regarding symptoms suggestive of acoustic neuroma thus promoting early diagnosis and successful treatment. The ANA publishes a quarterly newsletter, distributes patient information booklets, presents a biennial national symposium, promotes local support groups and maintains a library of information on acoustic neuroma.

Alexander Graham Bell Association for the Deaf
3417 Volta Place NW, Washington, D.C. 20007-2770
Voice: (202) 337-5220 Fax: (202) 337-8314 E-mail:agbell@aol.com

The Association is a nonprofit organization comprised of individuals who are hearing impaired, and their parents, professionals, and others. The organization's mission is to empower those with loss of hearing to function independently by promoting universal rights and optimal opportunities. They provide scholarships and awards to students and their families. They publish two periodicals, one research based, the other consumer oriented. There are over 20 chapters in North America, all of which provide leaflets on a range of problems affecting those suffering with hearing loss.

American Academy of Audiology [AAA]
8201 Greensboro Drive, Suite 300 McLean, VA 22102
Voice: (703) 610-9022 Toll-free: (800) 222-2336
Fax: (703) 610-9005 web:http://www.audiology.org

The Academy is a professional membership organization of audiologists. Their bimonthly journal publication provides audiologists with ongoing research knowledge. Their annual national meeting allows clinicians and scientists a forum for exchange and education in the areas of hearing science and hearing aids. They are not staffed for consumer outreach.

American Academy of Otolaryngology —Head and Neck Surgery, Inc.

One Prince Street, Alexandria, Va 22314
Voice: (703) 836-4444 TTY: (703) 519-1585 FAX (703) 683-5100
E-mail: entinfo@aol.com web:http://www.entnet.org

This organization was founded in 1896 as a medical specialty society. Its 11,000 members are physicians who provide medical care and surgery for disorders of the ears, nose and throat, head and neck regions. The primary missions of the Academy are to provide continuing medical education and to represent the interests of the specialty in governmental areas.

The Academy publishes about a dozen patient education leaflets on various aspects of hearing loss which are available to the public at no charge. They also will refer you to a local practitioner if you specifically request the "Physicians List."

American Speech-Language-Hearing Association [ASHA]

10801 Rockville Pike, Rockville, Maryland 20852
Consumer Hotline: (800) 638-8255 Fax: (301) 571-0457
Voice: (301) 897-5700

ASHA is the national professional, scientific and credentialing association for audiologists and speech-language pathologists. Their mission is to ensure that all people with speech, language or hearing disorders have access to quality services to help them communicate more effectively. Working toward this goal, ASHA awards the Certificate of Clinical Competence (CCC) to audiologists and speech-language pathologists who meet strict requirements. They accredit master's-level education programs and clinical service programs which meet their standards. They also inform the public about communication disorders through materials available by request. They will also make referral to a provider in your area.

American Tinnitus Association
P.O. Box 5, Portland, OR 97207
Voice: (503) 248-9985 Fax: (503) 248-0024
E-mail:tinnitus@ata.org

This nonprofit organization is dedicated to the support of scientific research leading to a better understanding of tinnitus. They provide pamphlets of information on tinnitus and publish a consumer-based quarterly magazine discussing various issues pertaining to understanding this problem.

Better Hearing Institute [BHI]
P.O. Box 1840, Washington, D.C. 20013
Voice: (703) 642-0580 Toll Free Helpline: (800) 327-9355
E-mail:mail@betterhearing.org web:http://www.betterhearing.org

BHI, a nonprofit educational organization, implements public information programs on hearing loss and available hearing solutions for millions with uncorrected hearing loss. The Institute promotes awareness of hearing loss and help through television, radio, and print media public service messages that typically feature well-known celebrities who themselves suffer from impaired hearing. You may contact them for literature on hearing loss or specific subjects such as tinnitus, hearing aids, children's ear conditions, lists of local hearing professionals, and assistive listening devices.

The Caption Center
125 Western Avenue, Boston, MA 02134
Voice/TTY: (617) 492-9225 Fax: (617) 562-0590
E-mail:caption@wgbh.org
In Los Angeles: 610 No. Hollywood Way, Suite 350, Burbank, CA 91505
Voice: (818) 562-3344 TTY: (818) 562-1919 Fax: (818) 562-3388
In New York: 475 Park Avenue South, 10th FL, NY, NY 10016
Voice: (212) 545-0854 TTY: (212) 545-8546 Fax: (212) 545-0957

The Caption Center is a nonprofit service of the WGBH Educational Foundation and the world's first television captioning agency. Captions translate the audio portion of a program or video, including dialogue, sound effects and off-screen voices, into a text on the screen. To view captions, consumers need either a television with a built-in decoder (mandatory in all sets sold since 1993), or a set-top decoder box.

Cochlear Implant Club International [CICI]
P. O. Box 464, Buffalo, New York 14223-0464
Voice/TTY: (716) 838-4662

This nonprofit organization was founded in 1981 by a small group of implant users in Nashville, Tennessee. Their original purpose was to help each other cope with the daily challenge of hearing impairment. Today, CICI has expanded to include adults, children, families, medical and professional counselors, educators and other interested individuals. CICI publishes a Newsletter, *Contact*, which provides readers with research information, developments in legislation and insurance coverage, personal experience stories, user tips, and news from various chapters.

The Education and Auditory Research [EAR] Foundation
2000 Church Street, Box 111, Nashville, TN 37236
Voice: (615) 329-7307 Voice/TTY
Toll Free: (800) 545-4327 Fax: (615) 329-7935

One of the mission's of the EAR Foundation is to administer education about Meniere's disease through their "Meniere's Network." This is a national network of people who share coping strategies regarding this condition. EAR publishes a few in-depth management brochures which provide education on Meniere's, including dietary management. They also publish a Newsletter, *Steady*, covering many aspects of the problems with Meniere's, and a Newsletter, *Otoscope*, which addresses problems more associated with hearing loss.

Hearing Education and Awareness for Rockers [HEAR]
San Francisco Center on Deafness
P.O. Box 460847, San Francisco, CA 94146
Voice: (415) 431-3277 24 Hr Hotline: (415) 773-9590 Fax: (415) 552-4296
E-mail:hear@hearnet.com web:http://www.hearnet.com

HEAR is a nonprofit public-benefit health organization founded in 1988. Their advisory board consists of some members—now hearing impaired—from a variety of the loudest 1960's Rock 'n Roll bands. The organization is dedicated to raising consumer awareness about the risks of noise, and its damaging effects on hearing. They've also produced a video on this subject for use in schools.You may contact them for a free leaflet about noise risks.

252

Hearing Health Magazine

Voice International Publications, Inc., P.O. Drawer V, Ingleside, TX 78362
Voice/TTY: (512) 776-7240 Fax: (512) 776-3278
E-mail:ears2u@hearinghealthmag.com
web:http://www.hearinghealthmag.com

Hearing Health's mission is simple: to educate and entertain people who are deaf or hard of hearing. Each issue (six per year) includes articles ranging from technological research and development, to humor, human success stories, and philosophical discussions about topics like education, cochlear implants, modes of communication, and living without hearing. You may contact them for a complimentary copy of a current magazine.

Hear Now

9745 East Hampton Avenue, Suite 300, Denver Co 80231-4923
Voice/TTY: (303) 695-7797 Consumer Hotline: (800) 648-4327 (V/TTY)
Fax (303) 695-7789 E-mail:107737.1272@compuserve.com

Hear Now is a national not-for-profit organization dedicated to making hearing accessible to very low income, hard-of-hearing people of all ages by providing hearing aids and cochlear implants. Entirely supported by private contributions, they have provided over 10,000 hearing aids to over 6,000 people and provided assistance with over 40 cochlear implants since 1992. They manage the only nationwide hearing aid recycling program, "Hear-O Program," which accepts all hearing aids, regardless of age or condition. You may contact them for more information or to request an assistance application.

HIP Magazine

1563 Solano Avenue, Suite 137, Berkeley, CA 94707
Voice: (510) 527-8993 Fax: (510) 523-4081
E-mail:folks@hipmag.org web:http://www.hipmag.org

This is a nicely oversized (11"x17") bimonthly magazine exclusively for children between ages eight and fourteen with hearing loss. It is nonprofit, with diverse sources of income, the principal being subscriptions. It is beautifully colorful with large attractive graphics which appeal to the kids, is educational and fun. No commercial advertising appears in it. Having begun in 1994 breaking just over 200 sales, they now tout over 7,000 paid subscriptions. They have won awards for excellence from the Parent's Choice Foundation and the Educational Press Association of America. Each issue contains a companion teaching guide with activities and ideas for parents and educators.

International Hearing Society [IHS]
20361 Middlebelt Road, Livonia, MI 48152
Voice: (248) 478-2610 Consumer Info: (800) 521-5247 Fax (248) 478-4520

The IHS began in 1951 as the primary organization for hearing aid dispensers. They conduct programs of competence qualification and training, and offer continuing education courses in the selection, fitting, counseling, and dispensing of hearing instruments. They also publish an industry magazine, the *Audecibel*, articles of which cover issues pertaining to hearing loss and hearing aid electronics, performance and use. A charitable subgroup of the IHS is the Hearing Aid Foundation which specifically focuses on education of the consumer. If you're looking for a board certified hearing instrument specialist (BC-HIS) in your area, the International Hearing Society can help you.

Job Accommodation Network [JAN]
918 Chestnut Ridge Road, P.O. Box 6080, Suite 1, Morgantown, WV 26506
Voice/TTY:Toll Free: (800) 526-7234 Fax: (304) 293-5407

This is an international consulting service that provides information about job accommodations, the employability of people with disabilities, and the removal of barriers as described by the Americans with Disabilities Act (ADA). If you have a disability, they will offer consulting services on how to modify your work setting, what assistive devices or methods you may need. They operate out of West Virginia University under a government grant through the President's Committee on Employment of People with Disabilities (which is listed separately in this chapter).

254

Lions Club
Lions Sight and Hearing Foundation
1016 North 32nd Street, Suite 1, Phoenix, AZ 85008
(602) 275-1764

Lions have a U.S. base of 170 nonprofit Clubs and have long been recognized for their worldwide financial assistance to those who could not afford corrective lenses or eye surgery. In addition, to pre-qualified candidates, they give hearing aids at no charge, and in some cases even ear surgery. Typically, such candidates are on a very low fixed income, don't own a home or car, and depend on subsidy assistance to get by (such as Social Security, Medicaid, Welfare, Disability, etc.). Their mission is to develop and use their own resources to enhance the lives of those less fortunate. You may also send them your old or broken and fractured hearing aids, salvageable parts of which are stripped and sent to foreign countries (particularly in South America) for re-assembly and donated to the poor.

National Association of the Deaf [NAD]
814 Thayer Avenue, Silver Springs, MD 20910-4500
Voice. (301) 587-1788 TTY: (301) 587-1789 Fax (301) 587-1791
E-mail:NADHQ@juno.com web:http://www.nad.org

This nonprofit association preserves and expands deaf awareness, deaf culture, and deaf heritage. Their primary areas of focus include grassroots advocacy and empowerment; captioned media; certification of sign language interpreters and American Sign Language and Deaf Studies professionals; deaf-related information and publications (including two periodicals: *The NAD Broadcaster*, and *The Deaf American Monograph*); legal advocacy; policy development and research; public awareness; and youth leadership development. They hold a biennial convention.

National Institute on Aging [NIA] -Information Center
P.O. Box 8057, Gaithersburg, MD 20898-8057
Voice. Toll Free: (800) 222-2225 TTY: (800) 222-4225 Fax (301) 589-3014

The NIA is responsible for the conduct and support of biomedical, social, and behavioral research, training, health information dissemination, and other programs with respect to the aging process and the diseases and other special problems and needs of the aged. They publish a number of detailed leaflets covering such broad areas as Aging, Grants, Diseases, Prevention, Medical Care, Medications, Planning for Later Years, and Safety.

National Institute on Deafness and Other Communication Disorders [NIDCD] -Information Clearinghouse
1 Communication Avenue, Bethesda, MD 20892-3456
Voice: (800) 241-1044 TTY: (800) 241-1055
E-mail:nidcd@aerie.com web:http://www.nih.gov/nidcd

This is a branch of the U.S. Government's National Institutes of Health. They are an information clearinghouse and can provide you with literature on various aspects of hearing loss if you call their toll free number, write, or contact their website. They have about 20 free brochures covering different areas of hearing problems.

Self Help for Hard of Hearing People, Inc. [SHHH]
7910 Woodmont Avenue, Suite 1200, Bethesda, MD 20814
Voice: (301) 657-2248 TTY: (301) 657-2249 Fax (301) 913-9413
E-mail:national@shhh.org web:http://www.shhh.org

SHHH seeks to provide information and educational outreach to people with hearing loss. Founded in 1979, their membership of 12,000 is the largest consumer organization in the world. Their extensive volunteer-based network includes 250 groups and chapters which reach an additional 9,500 hard of hearing people, their family members, friends, and others. They are governed by a 21-member volunteer board of trustees.

SHHH provides its educational offerings in a number of ways, including written materials such as the bimonthly magazine, *Hearing Loss: The Journal of Self Help for Hard of Hearing People*, and other publications and videos; annual conventions for consumers which exceeds 1,000 attendees; encouragement and participation in research activities with the government, private sector, and other nonprofit organizations; and the provision of guidance to national, state and local policy makers and private companies on a wide range of topics affecting people with hearing loss.

Silent News

133 Gaither Drive, Suite E, Mt. Laurel, NJ 08054-1710
Voice: (609) 802-1977 TTY: (609) 802-1978 Fax: (609) 802-1979
E-mail:SilentNews@aol.com

Silent News is a nonprofit company that publishes a monthly newspaper by the same name which focuses on all issues surrounding hearing loss and deafness. The average paper can exceed 50 pages, articles of which are quite varied. *Silent News* is divided into multiple sections consisting of Lifestyles, coverage on Sports, Editorial, Opinion, National and International News, Columnists, Letters to the Editor, Community Bulletin Board, Education News, Milestones, Special Report, Religion, Travel, People, Health and Crossword Puzzles.

INDEX

low frequency, 44
medical basis for evaluation of,
   165-166
myths of, 61-64
noise-induced, 58
non-aging factors of, 26
readiness for help with, 102-103
retiring with, 34-37
sensorineural, 111
types of, 45
Hear Now, 253
Hearing Review, The, 3
HIP magazine, 254
hyperacusis, 200. See *tinnitus*.

I

inner ear, (see *ear*).
International Hearing Society, 254

J

Job Accommodation Network, 254

L

labyrinthitis, 166-168. See *Meniere's
   Disease*.
Lions Club, 255
lipreading, (see *speechreading*.)
listening, 178-199
   active, 184
   easy situations of, 183
   in difficult situations, 187
   in large areas, 197-198
   practice of, 193-195
   taking control of, 199
   to native language, 187

M

Meniere's Disease, 58, 166-169, 204

N

National Association of the Deaf, 255

National Institute on Aging, 256
National Institute on Deafness and
   Other Communication Disorders
   [NIDCD], 256
noise, as a stressor, 222
   background, 51, 119, 125-126,
     156, 197
   from wind in hearing aids, 155
   hearing loss and, 119
   hunters and, 223, 225-226
   implications of, 222
   -induced hearing loss, 202, 214
   industrial, 26, 44, 226-227
   musicians and, 222, 226
   OSHA, 227-228
   Prevention of hearing loss from,
     222, 229
   Protection from, 226-227, 229
   recreational, 227
   risk, 224, 228.
   See *tinnitus*.
nursing homes, 40-41
   otoacoustic emissions, 205, 216-
     217

P

presbycusis, 22-24, 58
professional resources, 248-257

R

ringing in the ears, (see *tinnitus*.)

S

Self Help for Hard of Hearing People
   [SHHH], 256
signal processing, 84-85
Silent News, 257
sound, decibels of, 47
   frequency of, 48, 50
   intensity of, 47-48
   spectrum of, 51
   speed of, 46
   transmission of, 51
   vibrations of, 46, 48-49

THE CONSUMER HANDBOOK ON

HEARING LOSS & HEARING AIDS
THIS BRIDGE TO HEALING CAN CHANGE YOUR LIFE

"...A must read....The pearls of wisdom you harvest...will last a lifetime."
-Robin L. Holm, BC-HIS, Senior Editor, *Audecibel*

"I wish this had been available years ago!"
-Paula Bonillas, Editor, *Hearing Health Magazine*

"...The authors bring a wealth of experience and expertise..."
- David Kirkwood, Editor-in-Chief, *The Hearing Journal*

"Much in this book will prepare you for your journey toward better hearing."
-Karl Strom and Marjorie Skafte, Editors, *The Hearing Review*

"This book reveals that hearing loss is not insurmountable!"
-Donna L. Sorkin, Executive Director, Self Help for Hard of Hearing People (SHHH)

A quiet path is charted on how to achieve life satisfaction despite less than optimal hearing. A recurrent theme of pushing through the resistance gently and sensitively comes through. You'll understand how to align your expectations with actual hearing ability. This book is written for consumers with loss of hearing and their families. It addresses the whole person, not merely one aspect of the problem.

Clinical Audiologist Richard Carmen has been writing consumer books and articles on hearing loss for more than 20 years. In this one-of-a-kind book he brings together the most renowned U.S. audiologists, scientists and authorities, each seasoned professionals in their respective hearing specialty, and some who themselves have hearing loss and use hearing aids. What you'll read inside is state of the art.

- EXPLORE THE VOLATILE EMOTIONS AND ISSUES SURROUNDING HEARING LOSS
- LEARN WHERE AND HOW TO FIND HELP
- RECOGNIZE UNIQUE SITUATIONS AND REQUIREMENTS THAT COME WITH AGE
- TAKE A SELF-ASSESSMENT TEST AND FIND OUT IF YOU REALLY HAVE A PROBLEM
- UNCOVER WHY SOME PEOPLE REJECT HEARING AIDS BUT HOW THEY CAN WORK FOR YOU
- STUDY THE NUTS AND BOLTS OF HEARING AID MAINTENANCE AND THEIR LONGEVITY
- READ QUESTIONS/ANSWERS POSED TO 10 TOP EXPERTS
- MASTER INCREDIBLY EASY TECHNIQUES TO IMPROVE YOUR LISTENING AND HEARING ABILITY
- IDENTIFY CAUSES OF RINGING IN THE EARS
- INVESTIGATE NOISE AND DRUG EFFECTS ON HEARING, AND THEIR PREVENTION
- DISCOVER FABULOUS DEVICES BESIDES HEARING AIDS THAT SOLVE HEARING PROBLEMS

ISBN 0-9661826-0-X

51895>

9 780966 182606